GENERATION XL

Raising Healthy, Intelligent Kids in a
High-Tech, Junk-Food World

D1444288

GENERATION XL

Raising Healthy, Intelligent Kids in a
High-Tech, Junk-Food World

DR. JOSEPH MERCOLA
AND DR. BEN LERNER

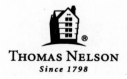

THOMAS NELSON
Since 1798

NASHVILLE   DALLAS   MEXICO CITY   RIO DE JANEIRO

Every commercially reasonable effort has been made to make this book as accurate as possible. The purpose of this book is to educate, and it represents the opinion of the authors. It is a review of scientific evidence available at the time the book was written and is presented for information purposes only. No individual or physician should use the information in this book for self-diagnosis, treatment, or justification in accepting or declining or providing any medical therapy for any health problems or diseases. Any application of the advice herein is at the reader's own discretion and risk. Therefore, any individual with a specific health problem or who is taking medication should first seek advice from his personal physician or healthcare provider before starting a nutrition program. The authors, authors' companies, and Thomas Nelson, Inc. shall have neither liability nor responsibility to any person or entity with respect to loss, damage, or injury caused or alleged to be caused directly or indirectly by the information contained in this book. Each clinical story has been significantly changed as to place, person, and sex in order to protect the individuals concerned. Any similarity to any individual case is purely coincidental. The names and trade names of products and businesses discussed in this book are for editorial, reference, and informational purposes only. The authors, authors' companies, and Thomas Nelson, Inc. are not affiliated with or sponsored by the manufacturers of such products.

Published in Nashville, Tennessee, by Thomas Nelson, Inc.

Thomas Nelson, Inc. titles may be purchased in bulk for educational, business, fund-raising, or sales promotional use. For information, please e-mail SpecialMarkets@ThomasNelson.com.

Library of Congress Control Number: 2007920303

ISBN-10: 0-7852-2186-7 (hardcover)
ISBN-13: 978-0-7852-2186-9 (hardcover)
ISBN-13: 978-0-8499-6493-0 (TP)

Printed in the United States of America

12 13 14 15 16 QW 6 5 4 3 2 1

CONTENTS

PREFACE
Taking a Stand for the Health of Our Children

As a doctor, a husband, and a father, when I look around at the way society currently works, I'm quite certain something is very wrong. All you have to do is look at the current levels of depression and obesity in both kids and adults, the epidemic levels of lifestyle-induced diseases, the increase in learning disorders, and the erosion of the family unit, and it becomes increasingly evident that the way we take care of ourselves and interact is not in the plan for what it takes to create health, peace of mind, and children who will grow to thrive in society.

Sit back for a moment and consider what is best for the health and development of the mind and body of a child. Quickly, you will see a problem.

Mind

We are born to nurture and develop imagination, concentration, adaptability, and planning. All of life and fulfillment requires creativity, strategy, relationships, a sense of humor, flexibility, and focus. These things are developed through adventure, investigation, crafts, art, reading, journaling, social interaction, physical activity, problem solving, and all that makes up real-life experiences.

All of these basic necessities of mental function and development have one thing in common: *none of them occur while watching TV or playing a video game.* In fact, the TV and video games do it *for* you, thus ensuring underdevelopment of mental function. Studies show that there is a direct correlation between time in front of a TV or computer screen and lowered IQ.

Organizations such as America's Foundation for Chess and Talaris Research

Institute are fighting to change this. By giving children an activity that requires actual brain activity, strategic planning, and thinking ahead, they are finding that children from impoverished situations are seeing success in their lives and their futures despite their circumstances. I fear that those who are in the best of circumstances are being put at risk, as they are often the ones who can afford the very technologies that could impair their future.

A great mind game for rebuilding cognitive function and imagination that have been diminished by technology is to play tic-tac-toe without a piece of paper.

From top to bottom:

Row 1: A1 (upper left corner), A2 (center left), and A3 (lower left)
Row 2: B1 (upper mid), B2 (center), B3 (lower mid)
Row 3: C1 (upper right corner), C2 (center mid), C3 (lower right)

You then play tic-tac-toe by calling out your move by the place in the grid rather than writing it down. Players are forced to remember their and their opponent's placements in addition to planning their next move. Since you or your children may not have used your brain in a while, it could cause pain and even soreness!

Body

As with the mind, we've poisoned the body. The food industry cranks out commercial after commercial selling all sorts of blue, green, or purple sugared cereals; artificial, easy-to-use, quick-to-make food items endorsed by a cartoon character or teen idol; and the latest gimmick to drive you to McDonald's, Burger King, or some other fast-food restaurant.

Childhood is a pivotal time for good nutrition. A child's cells and organs are growing at light speed and using nutrients in order to do so. While kid food is typically strange-colored or fast food, there's no more dangerous time to consume such things than when you're a child. Most people would think the sick, the elderly, and those with bad cholesterol need to be more careful with what they eat. But, as we're finding out fast, the problems we face today start with a Big Mac and a Pop-Tart as a kid. Organs and blood streams nurtured with junk food do not create the kind of foundation that will allow you to experience good health and longevity as an adult.

Kids were born to move, to kick, to jump, to leap, and to fall off swing sets and out of trees. Nowadays, the only kicking, jumping, leaping, and falling happening on a regular basis is being performed by the action figures on the TV or video-game screen. This inactivity creates not only obesity but poorly developed muscles, joints, and ligaments. Arthritis, spinal degeneration, and other joint and muscle dysfunctions once reserved for the aged are now being seen in children.

As children riddled with pain, illness, learning disorders, and even depression begin to show up everywhere, rather than looking at brain development, nutrition, and lack of movement as the culprits and doing what we can to begin producing health and well-being, concerned parents are turning to more and more medications. Think about that. Is that how we were designed? To make medication a way of life and to be drugged early on a consistent basis? What does the future hold for us when kids are overweight, out of shape, and taking medications for the effects? What kind of children are we creating? Those are the questions I ask myself every day in my home, in my Maximized Living Health Center in Celebration, Florida, and when I'm teaching doctors, leaders, and parents all over the country. These are the questions this book answers.

This is not a diet book; far, far from it. Dropping the next diet book into the same culture will do nothing but take up more room on your shelf. This is a call to begin looking at the way we now live our lives and the most cutting-edge information available today on how to simply and practically change it. We will show you how kids were created to eat, breathe, sleep, run, and live. At the same time we will help you change your family culture and recognize where the culture around you isn't working so you can avoid it or help to change it with us. Let other kids be a statistic, but not yours. Let other kids lead lives far below their potential, but not yours. Let your kids be everything you hoped they would be . . . and more.

The great part is, there's help. If you're overwhelmed, there are health professionals who are equipped to help and information designed to make it easier, not harder, to raise well kids. Any time you need to speak to someone during the course of reading this book, you can go to www.maximizedliving.com, and it will direct you to a trained healthcare provider in your area.

INTRODUCTION
Excelling in an Average World

Halfway through the twentieth century, the media riveted our attention on a national crisis that had reached epidemic proportions, a disturbing trend captured under the catchall phrase "Why Johnny Can't Read." Educators and parents scrambled to correct the problem of children advancing through school barely able to read. Today that urgent national question is "Why isn't Johnny (or Jenny) healthy and fit?" In this fast-food, high-tech, high-stress world, how can a child *excel rather then become XL*?

While no one was watching, several insidious trends quietly took hold in our culture over the past thirty years—things like profound inactivity, diets of supersized fast food and sugar-laden beverages, and whole generations of children addicted to television and video games. As we mad-dashed our way through the 1980s, 1990s, and early 2000s, American kids gained weight, leading to collective statistics that show no sign of abating unless we take drastic measures:

- One in every four American children are seriously overweight or at risk of becoming overweight. (An April 2006 report by the World Health Organization [WHO] showed that according to their new growth standard, 20 to 30 percent more young children may be overweight than previously thought when compared to the existing U.S. standard.[1])

- As other cultures such as Canada, Australia, and many European cities have now taken on a more Westernized lifestyle, they, too, are seeing a startling increase in childhood obesity.

- In the United States, 30 percent of boys and 40 percent of girls are at risk for developing type 2 diabetes—an obesity-related condition—sometime in their lives. In the 1990s, type 2 diabetes accounted for 8 to 45 percent of all new pediatric cases of diabetes—compared to fewer than 4 percent before the 1990s.[2]

- Obesity-related annual hospital costs for children more than tripled over two decades, from $35 million in the period from 1979 to 1981 to $127 million in the period from 1997 to 1999.[3]

- Overweight children are at risk of developing serious emotional and psychosocial problems due to society's harsh view of obesity.[4]

- Over the past three decades, childhood obesity has more than doubled for preschool children (two to five years old) and adolescents (twelve to nineteen) and more than tripled for children ages six to eleven years.[5]

- By fourteen years of age, 32 percent of girls and 52 percent of boys consume three or more eight-ounce servings of sweetened soft drinks daily.[6]

- Children's use of media (television, video games, radio, cassette/CD players, VCRs, and computers) averages five and one-half hours a day, with eight- to eighteen-year-olds racking up more than six and one-half hours daily.[7]

Almost everyone agrees that the obesity epidemic started around the early 1980s. According to Katherine Flegal, an epidemiologist at the National Center for Health Statistics, the percentage of obese Americans stayed relatively constant through the 1960s and 1970s at 13 to 14 percent and then spiked by 8 percentage points in the 1980s. By the end of that decade, nearly one in four Americans were obese.[8]

That steep rise, which continued through the 1990s, is the single most astounding feature of the epidemic. Any theory that tries to explain obesity in America has to account for that. Meanwhile, *overweight children nearly tripled in number.*[9] And for the first time, physicians began diagnosing type 2 diabetes in adolescents. Type 2 diabetes often accompanies obesity. It used to be called adult-onset diabetes, but now, for the obvious reason, it is not.

Poor nutrition, being unfit, and gaining weight aren't just problems in and of themselves. They reduce quality of life, change emotional states, affect learning, lower immunity, and lead to and/or contribute to the development of a host of other related disorders in children. While obesity has been on the rise, nearly all childhood conditions have increased exponentially right along with it. Learning disorders and hyperactivity, allergies, infections, asthma, and mental illness have all risen at alarming rates.[10—15]

If you are a parent with a child under the age of eighteen, this book could be your clarion call to action on an issue you cannot afford to ignore. Since prevention is always easier (and wiser) than cure, incorporating the lifestyle changes suggested in this book will give your child a realistic way to reach and maintain a healthy weight, dramatically reduce his or her risk of developing type 2 diabetes, cardiovascular disease, and other health risks, and build a strong body and positive mental attitude.

Whether or not your child appears healthy and fit to you right now, the principles for creating a healthy lifestyle can and should be applied to every child regardless of appearance. And while some children's metabolism levels will keep them from gaining weight, other visible and invisible problems—such as learning disorders, hyperactivity, depression, acne, frequent illness, stunted growth, arteriosclerosis, failure to succeed, and more—can result from unhealthy eating and lack of exercise. It's also important to note that children can be at a normal weight or even underweight for years and then suddenly add weight in the teen years, when making a change in eating habits can be much more difficult.

The underlying message of this book is that healthy living, healthy eating, and exercising aren't just for overweight kids. Please don't make this potentially lethal assumption! The effects of poor diet and a sedentary lifestyle are a national emergency—one we cannot put off addressing any longer. As a parent, your role is critical not only for this generation but for generations to come.

The Parent Trap

Physical and emotional problems in American children have increased exponentially over the last several decades. Yet, now that we've arrived at this alarming state, a curious phenomenon is taking place: parents of overweight, unfit, unhealthy children usually fail to recognize that their children have a problem.

Even more dumbfounding is that among parents of severely obese children, only 3 percent believe their child is overweight, and 8 percent actually think their child is *underweight!* The remaining majority—by a large percentage—believe their child's weight is normal.[16]

The facts above are a real wake-up call that parents do not have their feet planted in reality. It is hard to believe that only one in twenty parents of severely overweight children would consider their children overweight, and harder still to believe that nearly one in ten consider them to be underweight! As a society we are so accustomed to seeing overweight children that we don't see the problem even when it is happening right before our eyes, in our own homes. Perhaps this shouldn't come as a surprise in a nation of steadily increasing waist-lines—parents often deny their own obesity, making it easy for them to overlook it in their kids.

Do you find yourself making these common excuses about your child's health and weight problems?

- She doesn't like healthy food, and I feel guilty forcing it on her.

- I don't have time to prepare healthy meals—fast food is so much easier in our hectic world, not to mention cheaper.

- He loves his video games (television programs, etc.) and has never been the athletic type.

- Little trips to Dairy Queen are rewards for good behavior—I don't want to take away that incentive.

- She's so addicted to soft drinks I could never get her to start drinking water—plus, I like drinking them myself.

- He seems like a normal kid to me—why be so hard on him?

- Girls often "plump up" before puberty. Her body will trim down on its own in the next few years.

- He inherited "fat genes" and there's nothing I can do about it. Everyone in our family is overweight.

How did you score? If you found yourself agreeing with even one of the above excuses, this book is for you. If you can relate to two or more, we urge you to take the first step toward creating healthy lifestyle changes for your child, starting today.

Suppose you hired a contractor to build your dream house. He comes highly recommended, and his rates are reasonable. Excited about seeing your dream come true, you sign the contract and hire the builder to create your dream house. However, as the weeks go by you notice an unsettling trend: Instead of using the quality building products he promised to use, the contractor substitutes them with cheaper alternatives (in an effort to "cut corners," he says apologetically). The foundation is not poured correctly and begins to crack before the framing goes up. It turns out the ground was not properly leveled on the building site, and that leads to even more problems. The wiring has to be redone, the paint has been thinned to make it stretch farther, and shoddy workmanship is evident throughout the house, from crooked doorways to improperly installed appliances. The end product is a house far inferior to the one you dreamed of, a house far short of its potential—and one you may even be ashamed of. Everything looked so good at the blueprint stage. What went wrong?

The answer to that question is obvious. Poor materials were substituted for quality ones; expert craftsmanship was sacrificed to poor workmanship. Like the adage says, "Garbage in, garbage out." What goes into the building of a house determines the quality of that house. Likewise, what goes into the building of a body and mind determines the health and stability of that body and mind. Is it any wonder American kids today, as a group, stack up so poorly to their European counterparts in terms of health and weight?

In many of those countries, where people frequently walk to nearby destinations rather than rely on cars, physical activity is built into the daily routine—it's just what you do. The availability of fast food is a lot less prevalent also, tipping the scale much more in favor of healthy diets.

Contrast that with America, where we supersize our fast-food meals, and one in every four drinks consumed is a soft drink. Our annual soda consumption averages out to more than fifty-six gallons for every man, woman, and child, amounting to more than $60 billion a year in sales. Can you believe the average girl eats one ounce of sugar and the average boy two ounces of pure sugar every day from sodas? That is nearly fifty pounds of sugar every year just from soft drinks. And this is *average*. Consider this statistic: for every can or glass of soda or sugar-sweetened beverage a child drinks, their obesity risk jumps 60 percent . . . not to mention the impact sugar has on physical and emotional well-being.[17]

If a child is out of shape and having trouble with his or her weight, there are only a few major causes:

- Inactivity (watching television and playing video games rather than playing outside to get exercise)

- Drinking soda and juice instead of water

- Eating sugar, bread, cereal, and other highly processed grains

Fortunately, while it may seem impossible at times, something can be done to prevent children (and adults) from being unhealthy, out of shape, unfit, or actually obese—or even completely reverse the process. The future health of our country is clearly related to having our children eat healthily and get moving. It is equally important that we invest time and energy in cultivating learning and relationship skills in our children—teaching them to dream, interact with others, and set goals rather than waste away in front of a TV or computer screen. As a parent, you are in a powerful position to influence your child toward a life of good, healthy habits. You are truly the key component in controlling childhood obesity.

The patterns you incorporate in your child's life could prevent a lifetime of chronic disease and emotional suffering. Fortunately or unfortunately, habits, thought patterns, and self-image developed in childhood have a strong chance of "sticking" well into adulthood. And don't forget the important role of modeling good behavior—your kids are watching *you* to see if you practice what you preach. If they see you reach for an apple instead of a doughnut, they are likely to do the same. If they see you go for a walk or shoot some hoops, they may catch the enthusiasm for exercise and join in. Similarly, if you are one who reads, responds well to stress, or is good at managing your time, it's likely you will breed the same habits into your children.

Any successful undertaking requires a realistic assessment of your starting point so you can arrive at your intended outcome. Otherwise the blueprint would be useless. So before we tackle the issue of preventing and reversing childhood obesity in the following pages, it's important to ask: How did we get here? Where did America go so wrong regarding the health—weight—outlook of its children?

A Vanishing Childhood

If you were a child of the mid-1970s or earlier, chances are your childhood was very active. A typical summer day may have looked something like this: You wake up, run downstairs, and eat a bowl of hot oatmeal or scrambled eggs and toast your mom made. After breakfast you go outside to find your friends and pick up where you left off playing ball in the vacant lot the day before. After three hours of softball, you head home for a sandwich and homemade soup. You get your household chores done, then meet your best friend for a hike through the woods behind your house. You're building a secret fort, so both of you spend the afternoon hauling scraps of lumber and a few necessary tools to "the spot." The afternoon flies by, and before you know it you hear your mom's dinner bell ring in the distance. After supper, the neighborhood kids gather to catch lightning bugs—the boys cavorting and turning cartwheels on the lawn to impress the girls. Finally, exhausted, but your body tingling with the vigor of youth, you bathe (if your mom makes you) and fall into bed for a night of deep, replenishing sleep.

One writer put it this way: "Open your window on a sunny afternoon, and what do you hear? The chirping of singing birds? The yelling of playing children? Odds are these days that you'll hear the birds but not the children. As kids spend more time in front of television, computer and video screens, their physical activity levels have decreased. And their body weights have increased."[18]

Sad but true. As Americans embraced the technology boom of the last third of the twentieth century, we forgot to factor one very critical component into the equation: less exercise (times multiple years) equals steady weight gain. Someone once said the price we pay for laborsaving devices is our local gym membership. Now we have to plan exercise into our days—and often even pay for it—or watch our bodies grow soft and flabby.

While America embraced new technology—and especially entertainment technology such as television and video games—kids grew more accustomed to staying inside to kill aliens on a screen rather than to running around and killing imaginary aliens in their backyards. After-school TV shows captivated a whole generation of young Americans, and the television often stayed on well into the evening hours. It's not uncommon for kids (and adults) to munch on unhealthy snacks while zoning out in front of the tube, compounding their sedentary stance with empty, fat-producing calories.

Several other trends gained a foothold on American youth as the clock ticked toward the millennium:

- Increasing portion sizes at fast-food chains and restaurants

- A dramatic spike in soft-drink consumption

- School cafeterias offering inexpensive junk food contrasted to the "hot square meal" of yesteryear

- The use of high-fructose corn syrup to sweeten and thicken "bland" foods

- TV commercials and other junk-food ads aggressively targeting children

- American children experiencing a simultaneous mental and emotional downward spiral

- The elimination of mandatory PE classes in many U.S. cities and states

We live in what Kelly Brownell, a Yale psychologist, calls a "toxic food environment" of cheap fatty food, large portions, pervasive food advertising, and sedentary lives. By this theory, as one article rendered it, "we are at the Pavlovian mercy of the food industry, which spends nearly $10 billion a year advertising unwholesome junk food and fast food."[19]

Taken all together these lifestyle and eating changes have exacted a heavy toll on American children. As parents, educators, medical practitioners, and policy changers, we owe it to our children to give them a vibrant, successful future and a healthy, wholesome, invigorating youth. How to go about that mission is the subject of this book. By following the precepts for health in this book, your child will learn how to:

- build her body's immune system to its peak levels to prevent major diseases and common illnesses;

- reach his optimal weight—while being satisfied by eating—and maintain his optimal weight for life;

- prevent the underlying causes of premature aging;

- boost daily energy and mental clarity;

- improve emotional well-being and outlook on life;

- help eliminate the underlying causes of conditions such as diabetes, heart problems, chronic fatigue, allergies, and much more; and

- maximize her IQ, have her best chance for success, and optimize her athletic performance.

Like anything else of true worth in life, achieving real health and optimal weight for your child is ultimately your (and their) decision. It's not uncommon to hear people wish they were healthier, leaner, and had more energy, and in the next breath complain that taking the steps toward achieving those goals is "too costly" or "too time-consuming." It's really a matter of getting priorities straight and remembering that your children have just one life to live.

As you read through this book, keep in mind these two important points: *First, avoid becoming overwhelmed with all the useful information*—in other words, avoid biting off more than you (or your child) can chew. Some people, when they encounter all the dietary and lifestyle changes required for optimal health and weight, become discouraged because they believe they have to make them all happen at once. *Second, don't become overmotivated and try to make all the changes happen at once.* Both approaches frequently lead to failure. The key with the insights in this book—and adopting positive changes in any aspect of your life—is to implement them in manageable bites. That means establishing a plan for your child over time and implementing the changes in phases into their life.

Chapter 10, "Making Changes That Stick," will help you by providing a simple approach and key reminders you can use to prioritize and build your child's "manageable bites" plan. Remember—you don't have to do it all at once, and every step you take is a step in the right direction.

We won't lie and tell you that making healthy choices is easy; it's not. It will always be easier to grab a Big Mac at the McDonald's drive-up window than to prepare a healthy meal. It's easier to slump on the couch watching TV next to your kids than to drive to the park for a game of tag football. But those healthy choices are infinitely worth the effort. We trust that you'll make that effort on behalf of your children—who are the world's future in the truest and most abiding sense of the word—and also on behalf of yourself, because once you begin making changes you'll understand how fulfilling this new way of life can be.

CONFESSIONS OF A TWINKIE-EATING TV JUNKIE

1

Picture for a moment a scene from a 1970s sitcom: a Cleveland suburb with typical middle-class neighborhoods of large, treed lawns and dual-parent homes. So far so good. Inside one house are a father, mother, and three boys. The oldest boy, sporting a red afro and plaid pants, is about nine years old. As he sits on the sofa beside his siblings, munching a Twinkie, his eyes glaze over from the bluish glare of the TV parked across the room. In fact, if you take a closer look, you'll see that all five family members are busy eating some kind of sugary snack while zoning out in front of the tube—a scene repeated virtually every night in this household.

That redheaded boy is me, Ben Lerner. I wasn't always the co-founder of Maximized Living; I was born into a family whose main entertainment was eating. Although I grew up in Ohio, my family life was deeply entrenched in the long-standing culture of Queens, New York, where I was born and my extended family had lived for years. Everything revolved around food. It was our main pastime and our reward for everything. Two or three times a week we went over to somebody's house with a little white bakery box for a social call. We literally lived off New York-style pizza, cheesecake, and whatever was in those little white boxes. For breakfast, my brothers and I downed bowls of Fruity Pebbles or Cap'n Crunch. If we were going to have fun, it usually involved food.

I was never heavy as a kid, but my horrible diet led to all the typical child health problems times ten. Constantly fighting sore throats, colds, and joint problems, I got to know the inside of my doctor's office a little too well. If Ritalin were as popular back then as it is today, I would have been forced to

1

walk the school halls with a Ritalin IV drip. The only reason I didn't have a weight problem was that I was active in a way many kids aren't today. During the summer I'd often get on my bike and head down to a friend's house for all-day football. Even though I was active, I was still putting in a good forty hours a week in TV time, and the legacy of my family was always hanging over my head. In the Lerner family, every adult I knew was overweight and lived a sedentary life. It was a fate promised to me as well. I remember standing on the fourth step of our home in Mayfield Heights, Ohio, when my mother said to me, "When you're thirty, you're going to be fat like the other men in the family." I looked at her and said, "You know, Mom, Billy's mom said he was going to be an astronaut when he grew up."

That's right, while other kids were being told they could be lawyers and presidents when they were older, I was being told I was going to have big pants. It was my birthright—all I had to do was look at the evidence all around me.

Destined for Bigness?

Seeing my destiny spelled out in longer and longer belts, I started to get a little worried. I knew food was a problem; I knew my parents, friends, and relatives weighed too much. I just didn't know what in the world to do about any of it. After all, for years I'd eaten whatever I wanted whenever I wanted, just like the rest of my family, without ever once thinking about the consequences.

Sound familiar? I was raised on the three C's: Cow products, Chemicals, and empty Calories. At the time I thought there were only two major food groups: Fruity Pebbles and pepperoni pizza. If it wasn't loaded with artificial colorings, flavorings, or a list of ingredients even my science teacher couldn't pronounce, I didn't eat it. I certainly didn't feel unique. I was part of a generation raised on frozen dinners, snacks from 7-Eleven, and a revolutionary way of eating that was spreading across the country as quickly as backsides were spreading across the car seats we were all suddenly eating in: fast food.

My parents were always on diets. My dad would lose as much as one hundred pounds and then gain it all back, something I now know to be extremely dangerous. Sadly, they did not possess knowledge of how to eat healthfully or well. It was either starve or eat. We were always "on" or "off" a diet. I would go on the diets with my parents, and I started having concerns that I was heading in their footsteps. Though I was barely conscious of it, the first few times I

2

heard the phrase "you'll be fat too someday," I was already making internal commitments to buck the system. That internal nudge flickered into full-blown determination by the time I entered junior high.

While the family naysayers unwittingly propelled me toward wellness, something else added fuel to the fire burning inside me: the desire to fit in. Every adolescent kid worries about how well they fit in at school, but for some kids this teenage angst morphs into agony; the daily bus ride alone can be enough to make them want to walk.

Obviously, with everyone in my family being overweight, appearance was not at the top of the priority list. I was allowed to go to school looking unkempt, my curly red hair and plaid pants screaming *misfit*. I didn't understand what the deal was—as far as I knew you just needed pants and a shirt, right? So when I took my big red afro and plaid pants out into the community I couldn't understand why other kids didn't always accept me.

There's no question that those early days of trying to figure out who I was—and how I fit into the world—fueled my passion for succeeding. They provided the impetus for change. I made a conscious decision at age thirteen: "I'm not going to stay on this road; I'm not going to stay unpopular and weird. I can beat this; I can become accepted. I can become healthy and live a thinner life."

Sports, I decided, were my ticket to being cool. They also fell in line with my newfound pursuit of health and fitness. I was an amateur wrestler throughout junior high, high school, college, and for several years after college, honing my body by working out with weights and controlling my "weight class." I typically competed in a weight class that was fifteen or twenty pounds below my normal weight. During wrestling season, I sometimes had to "make weight" two or three times per week. As a result, I lived on and off a diet for nearly two decades—first from my parents' example and then from my own compulsion to succeed at wrestling.

A Weight-Loss Laboratory

While making weight was often nothing less than torture, the good part was that wrestling turned out to be a weight-loss laboratory for me.

All through junior and senior high, I was dieting in the dark. During those times, losing weight was extremely hard, and I endured a tremendous amount

3

of pain and suffering. When you are that young, you want to eat like an elephant, but I had to look like a gazelle—lean, muscular, fast, and hard to pin down. It wasn't until after several years of college that I finally learned to eat properly. After learning what to eat and when to eat it, I was able to lose even more weight than before, lose it faster, and actually eat twice as much food.

The results of my wrestling laboratory experiments showed me that eating well doesn't mean deprivation. Turning away from bad eating choices became its own reward as I saw and felt the changes within my body. A large part of being overweight, I now realize, is being poisoned and swollen from all the indigestible (man-made and/or altered) food stored as fat and fluids in your system. A lifetime of such eating takes its toll on any body. I only have to look as far as my own family for proof.

You see, I was named after my grandfather, whom I never met. Both of my grandfathers died of heart disease—in their fifties. My oldest uncle died in his fifties too. In fact, my passion for wellness today is rooted in tragedy: I watched my father die of a heart attack at age fifty-two and my mother suffer a stroke one year later. But even then, as a young man in my twenties, I knew my parents' poor health wasn't the result of a single problem, the need to diet. Taking care of yourself is complex. You need a plan for how to eat, how to cook, what to do at school or work, where, when, and how you will exercise, and how to do this as a family.

That quest for a holistic approach to sustainable health—what I call maximized living—propelled me first to major in nutrition and then to study chiropractic. In chiropractic I discovered a proven pathway to build health instead of merely treating disease. Seeing thousands of patients a year, I witnessed firsthand their frustration as they tried their hardest and yet failed to make the lifestyle changes they so desperately desired—especially weight loss. My desire to help people succeed in their own health quests led me to develop the simple, attainable, step-by-step methods that are the foundation for my professional practice, the Center for Maximized Living. The principles work, and you'll discover why and how in this book.

The Apathy and Denial of Obesity

Whenever I've studied and worked with kids who have weight or health problems, their feedback runs the gamut of responses. Some say, "That's just me;

I don't care." It kind of bothers them, but they dismiss it. I call this the apathetic response. When surveyed, nearly half of all obese people or parents of obese kids deny that being overweight will hurt them or their children. Others readily admit that the challenge of obesity or not fitting in leads to depression, which leads to more overeating or the habits that excluded them in the first place. For some (like me), feeling excluded serves as a good motivator to overcome the habits and choices that cause the rejection. Others may desire to change but simply do not know where to start—or how to make the changes stick.

We are all wired differently, with our own unique emotional and spiritual makeups. God created every human body with an innate inclination toward wholeness. Isn't that wonderful news? Your body yearns to be healthy!

Whether you are a parent, an educator, a health practitioner, or a school-age kid who battles with being fit, my desire is not to force change but to take you by the hand and show you how to take small, steady steps toward a life of wellness. Let me be the first to assure you that the principles found in this book—the same ones I built my practice on—produce results that are typical: safe, steady weight loss and a body built strong through good food and exercise.

Is There a Fat or a Sick Gene?

Growing up, I concluded that my family suffered from Poor Genetics Syndrome, or PGS. Rather than become discouraged, I vowed to overcome my PGS. I had to choose a completely different path through life—a path I now know everyone can follow. At forty, my cholesterol is one-third of what my father's was at this age, and my blood pressure is half.

Over the years of caring for the neurological and nutritional well-being of hundreds of thousands of people in my practice and serving as a chiropractor, nutritionist, and fitness trainer to the U.S. Wrestling Teams in six World Team competitions and two Olympics, I've discovered something that may come as a surprise to you: PGS is a myth. In our battle of the bulge, Americans consistently blame their genes as the chief culprit. However, I've seen super fit, healthy people with seemingly bad genes and overweight, sick people with what should have been great genes.

A common misconception is that some "lucky" people have high or "fast" metabolism, and some "unlucky" people have low or "slow" metabolism. Those who struggle with weight gain often lament that they were simply born with "bad glands," or PGS, but the reality is that the only glands involved here are usually the salivary glands.

We all have some genetic tendencies to be high-strung, low-strung, stomach-big, or heart-weak. However, these are just tendencies. They are not death sentences—or weight sentences—pronounced with finality over our lives. Tendencies can be overcome. While some people may have a genetic tendency to burn less caloric power and store more fat than others, in most cases the metabolism is caused to be low or high by the person themselves. The law of thermodynamics states that if a body burns more calories than it consumes, it will lose weight. And if a body consumes more calories than it burns, it will gain weight.

The truth about metabolism is that your body's efficiency at burning fat and calories is determined more by the way you and your child live your lives and less by your genetics. Movement, along with eating the right foods in the right amounts for your metabolic type (more on this later), all speed up or normalize the metabolism and cause the body to find or maintain its ideal weight.

What's Wrong with the Wellness Movement?

Over the past several years I've become increasingly bothered by something— if the number of wellness businesses and products is booming, why has being unhealthy and out of shape become such an epidemic? Granted, most wellness products are aimed at adults, not children, but this "wellness" trend still begs the question: If adults (including parents) are more aware of wellness issues now than at any other time in our nation's history, why are they allowing their children to make such poor health choices? The history of wellness dates all the way back to 1961 when Weight Watchers held its first meeting. Since then we've seen gyms pop up in every suburban shopping mall; Suzanne Somers's ThighMaster infomercials hit the airwaves in the eighties, Body by Jake and Tae Bo in the nineties, and South Beach, Atkins, and Dr. Phil's weight-loss plans started the new millennium.

What has been the result of the wellness revolution? We're bigger and more out of shape than ever. Obesity numbers have soared in the last two decades, tripling and even quadrupling for children and adults in the United States and abroad. Diseases related to obesity now kill more people than smoking and nearly every other kind of medical condition.[1]

While wellness businesses and products have made incredible advances over the last four decades, the actual wellness of the nation has retreated almost as quickly in the opposite direction. As we study other societies that continue to experience wellness while lacking the sophisticated tools we've created in the United States, it becomes evident health and fitness are not created by stuff; *they're created by culture.*

In our culture every adult and most children have cell phones; our schools now have McDonald's and Pizza Hut vendors; we can't imagine a week without stress or an unrushed moment. We demand fast service and instant relief; our bloodstreams are 75 percent Starbucks; we have a pill for every ill and a potion for every emotion. It's considered exercise if you have to do long math or compete in an intense game of Nintendo hockey. In this environment, chances are the next company, book, supplement, or exercise machine won't suddenly produce an army of healthy people.

Norms Are Really *Abnorms*

Cultures or societies contain norms. It seems that when it comes to health in America, however, what is a norm is always dangerously wrong.

For example, my practice is located across the street from a McDonald's. As much as we all know the dangers of that "food," the norm in America remains the same regarding fast food because the line there is always immense. In other words, norms are typically *abnorms.*

Therefore, if you want to become well, first you have to become free. Free from the typical way our culture lives.

What are some of the cultural abnorms in our lives that prevent us from becoming healthier, happier, and more well-adjusted people? The following are some abnorms worth rethinking.

Soft Drinks

The ingestion of soft drinks for kids ages six to seventeen has tripled over the course of the last three decades.[2] This is linked to the significant rise in weight of the average child due to adding a couple hundred calories a day from sugar.

Television

TV is where you receive the most misinformation about health issues, largely through commercials. If you do not think you're prone to the effects of commercials, see if you can answer these questions:

- What goes, "Plop, plop, fizz, fizz"?

- How do you spell relief?

- What's the nighttime "stuffy head fever so you can rest" medicine?

- What fast-food chain does it "your way"?

- What worldwide company encourages you to "Just do it"?

Medical Overutilization

One of the hardest pills for me to swallow is watching almost everyone swallowing pills. If you take a prescription or an over-the-counter medication every time you have sinus problems, allergies, a headache, a cold, the flu, an ache, a pain, or a sleeping problem, you are constantly putting toxins in the body and altering organ function and the normal immune response—thus, the "side effects" that are placed on *all* drug labels and ads. It's acceptable only because it's the norm.

Refined and Packaged Foods

With the motto "Quick, easy, tasty," it's easy to get lured into an abnormal life of convenient foods. However, when something comes out of a package, can, or machine it contains chemicals, hydrogenated oils, and sugar-based preservatives that cannot be broken down and are of no use to the body. These foods linger in the system and cause symptoms of poor health, affect your moods, create fatigue, rob the body of important nutrients, and shorten your life span.[3]

Not Using Natural Healthcare Methods

Sound nutritional programs, adequate supplementation, chiropractic care, fitness, and relaxation techniques are no longer *alternative* health care. They are *no-alternative* health care. In other words, there's no alternative to these things. If you skip them, your health suffers. For example:

- If someone is suffering from challenges related to poor diet, nutrient deficiency, food allergies, malabsorption related to nutrition, there's no alternative to finding a qualified nutrition expert to help.*

- If you or your child has postural abnormalities, scoliosis, or mal-alignment of the spine due to falls, traumas, or genetic factors, there's no alternative to choosing the right chiropractor and get this corrected and maintained.*

Until you change your thinking and move away from the "norms," history has shown nothing will change your wellness or that of your child. Where's the missing link in all this wellness frenzy? How can we make healthy changes that stick for a lifetime? Just keep reading.

Inspiration vs. Discipline

Have you ever noticed that people don't respond well to "have to" or "should" statements? Suppose you tell your sons and daughters they "have to" clean their rooms or they "should" eat every green bean on their plates. Their response is likely to be less than enthusiastic. Just the simple phrasing of "should" and "have to" alone is enough to call up a little rebellion in all of us. The reason why is obvious. "Have to" and "should" require discipline, and, like motivation, discipline ultimately runs short. What happens when we run out of willpower or "fall off the wagon" with our good intentions to eat more healthily and exercise more? We end up falling back into the same old poor-eating, not-exercising cycle. Now imagine the struggle your child will have if you as an adult find the challenge daunting!

There is a better way, for both you and your child, as you seek to incorporate healthy choices into your lives. Instead of committing to make changes out of true-grit determination (discipline), try changing the way you phrase your goals. If you failed at making healthy choices in the past, you may have concluded the problem is a lack of discipline. I would like you to change that phrase from "a lack of discipline" to "a lack of inspiration." People who are inspired to do something are able to transcend the mundane sense of "have to"

---

*For recommendations on healthcare professionals trained in nutritional testing and spinal correction, go to www.maximizedliving.com.

and find purpose and meaning behind their goals. Your child is a precious, one-of-a-kind gift from God with only one life to live. As you focus on that reality and how every choice made in the right direction brings you (and them) one step closer to a lifetime of wellness, your former "bootstrap mentality" will transform into inspiration.

Even if you permitted unhealthy eating habits and a sedentary lifestyle for your child in the past, remember that in the race of life it's the finish that counts. Your child may have gotten off to a rocky start and had a less-than-ideal middle, but they are still young enough to make changes that stick for life and carry them to a strong finish.

I often remind my clients that every one of us is a "work in progress." Think of your child as a construction zone. While his or her body and life may look as if it just got hit by a wrecking ball, remember that sometimes the old, worn-out structure has to be destroyed to make room for a brand-new building in its place.

Along with Dr. Mercola and the thousands of clients and patients we have helped, I am living proof that no such thing as an obesity curse, disease destiny, or PGS exists. By combining nutrition, exercise, and a lifestyle of balance, all the pieces of the puzzle come together to create wholeness and maximized living for your child, which is the goal of this book.

WHY PEER INFLUENCE IS SO POWERFUL

2

W e've enlisted the expertise of Dr. Em Twoey, author of *Proteen*[1] and a psychology professor at Palm Beach Atlantic College, to help understand the impact peers have on self-esteem, lifestyle choices, and physical well-being. Kids automatically group themselves into associations via sports, school classes, community clubs, church, youth groups—you name it. These peer groups are so predominant that it's rare to see the true loner, the kid who identifies with no one but himself. Kids rarely roam alone—especially as they grow into teenagers.

Being part of a positive peer group improves relationships and behaviors. Not surprisingly, kids who maintain close ties to their parents and other adults possess more confidence and better self-esteem. When those adult relationships involve accountability, kids demonstrate even higher levels of self-esteem. (Now you know why communication with your kids is so critical!)

A child who fits easily into his preferred peer group experiences less stress throughout the day—going to school, adjusting to classes, doing homework, participating in sports, resolving conflicts with friends, learning how to relate to the opposite sex, and so forth. No wonder peer groups play such a significant role in a child's level of happiness and satisfaction—and why rejection by peers can seem so damning.

Peers can also act as agents of change regarding questions about the future, adult roles, and social etiquette. And talk about the power of peers: Research shows that kids with negative behaviors often change for the better after participating in positive group activities. Suddenly, those same kids are more likely to feel better about themselves.

While better peer relationships foster more positive behaviors, this is only one side of the coin. Outward behavior has its place, but how do we foster the inner well-being of our kids? How do we enable them to feel good about themselves in a society where outward appearance is the only thing that is judged?

Looking on the Inside

Inner health or emotional well-being is the touchstone of identity. Deep inside all of us is an underlying need to feel good about ourselves. However, as we relate outwardly toward one another, this inner need is rarely met. Why? Because we often experience a "disconnect" between our desire for sincerity and our interactions with others. We don't want to appear vulnerable about our need for real sincerity. We're afraid people won't like us anymore if they see the real "us." Accepting this negative presupposition is the first step down the slippery slope toward a false self, causing us to behave in ways contrary to healthy self-awareness. So we exchange our true selves for fabricated facades of outward appearance.

This "social self" becomes the mask we wear anytime we interact with others. It keeps us safe—or so we reason. Kids do this all the time as they try to find their way into a peer group, whether it be the school football team, the drama club, or the "cool" clique. Kids want so much to fit in that they will conform to the group norm, whatever that may be. We see this dynamic at work even among negative peer groups such as street gangs. Birds of a feather flock together, and kids want to be accepted. Many teenage boys would rather be wanted for crime than not wanted at all.

So how do children and teens feel good about themselves on the inside while trying to be what they think their peers want? Our relationships often dictate that we sacrifice the former (emotional health) for the latter (acceptance by peers). Remember, kids want acceptance at any cost. They will move toward social acceptance in lieu of inner emotional health.

Here's where parents and other caring adults can step in, meeting that need for inner health and fostering self-esteem in their children. (Kids will relate to adults who take the time to talk with them, do not argue or preach, and communicate caring and understanding.) That sounds like a tall order for many parents, but it's the only way to foster open lines of communication. And communication is key to a healthy relationship with your son or daughter.

So what really is "self-esteem"? The word *self* in self-esteem is very misleading. This is because in today's culture, "self" has nothing to do with it. Who you decide you are is usually based on what others have given you the perception you are or what others have projected you to be.

When we are infants and toddlers, we assume we're loved. Therefore, we go around acting any way we please and demanding anything we want. Eventually, as we're judged by our appearance or personality, we begin to paint a self-image. Suddenly it may not be okay to be outgoing, expressive, charismatic, or to dance around. We begin to do what we should, ought, or must and what is necessary to be deemed acceptable to fit in or, in some cases, not be seen at all.

Based on this limited you, you make decisions and perform actions the rest of your life. The result is an outcome far less than your potential and a future that falls short of all you were born to be.

The other essential reason "self" has nothing to do with it is that our perceptions of ourselves are also greatly determined by our paternal and maternal figures. True self-worth comes from a feeling of being unconditionally loved. Unconditional love, the love that God has for you, is based not on your actions but on your core essence. Unfortunately, all too often it appears to us that our parents love us only for A's and B's or home runs and not for who we really are. This causes us to believe we are not valued for who we are, but for what we accomplish. Then, as we accomplish, it's still not enough. If we don't accomplish, we're worthless.

You can build a strong foundation in your children by continually expressing that they are valuable and loved just as they are. Help them to see their true worth when others neglect or reject them. The following are six specific things parents can do to help their kids feel good about themselves, using the acronym ELICIT:

1. Example

The first thing we all need to be is a good example. Kids will read your behavior and follow what you do more quickly than what you say. If kids see us indulging in inappropriate behavior, they will copy our bad habits. As parents, we must focus our attention on our kids and make them our first priority. We must be examples. This is especially critical in the teen years, because our sons and daughters are becoming the persons they will be for the next few years—young adults. Modeling healthy ways of relating to others will enable them to do the same.

Again, we won't lie and tell you this is easy. Being a good example takes a tremendous amount of effort, especially in light of all the forces competing for our kids' attention. This inner need for security is critically important but very difficult to access. Kids learn to guard their true needs through defense mechanisms; they have to know they can trust us.

If your child is a teen, remember that the psychological defenses peak during these moody years. It will take time and loving persistence to break through these defenses.

Be an example to your kids; they are starving for attention from good people.

2. Love

Don't just love; love your child with affection. The need for love and closeness is as strong as any physical need, and the best place to get it is in the home. We've all heard about the devastating consequences for babies who are deprived of love. Older kids are no different. They need love and affection too, and if they don't get it at home they will find it in the arms of someone else. For teens, this deep-seated desire for love may lead to a life of promiscuity, where they literally look for love in all the wrong places. Many teens are willing to trade sex for love, or they confuse sex with love.

Loving our kids with affection nudges them toward emotional health as they grow into adulthood.

3. Irritation

Although kids can be annoying, try to avoid becoming irritated by the things they do. Irritation is the opposite of affection: while affection builds emotional attachments with our kids, irritation weakens them. Affection bonds; irritation separates—and produces insecure, resentful teenagers.

Irritation is exactly what the dictionary tells us it is—something that causes an inflammation, an annoyance, or provocation. When irritated by their kids, many parents mistakenly use that opportunity to punish or discipline their children. We are not talking about misbehavior here but rather an attitude that says, "You are less than adequate; you have not reached my expectations."

Kids are perceptive. If they pick up on the message that we find them irritating, they internalize the belief that they will never live up to our standards. How many people have spent their entire lives trying to please an intolerant parent? Total acceptance is the only way to go. When kids know they will not be condemned, the power of love works a miracle, creating emotional, inner peace.

4. Compassion

Kids need to know that we approve of every aspect of their lives—even the way they wear their hair. Seriously, is their green hair or black clothing a good yardstick for measuring their self-worth? Compassion shows acceptance and approval of all areas of your child's life. The point is not to attach acceptance to looks. Their appearance, abilities, and habits all need approval from us.

What does your child do well? Tell him about it! Praise her for her efforts, even if they are less than stellar at times. A level of competence in any area is not the criterion for acceptance. If we are comfortable with ourselves, then we can accept our children. Once we communicate our compassion toward our kids, we can then lovingly help them overcome any weaknesses.

5. Interest

Really listening to someone conveys interest on your part. It says you care. It also conveys that the person talking is of value to you. As a parent, you're in a great position to practice the skill of listening and learn how to be an active listener. Here are three simple steps to help you become a better listener:

Step One. Be open and nonjudgmental. Kids need someone to listen to them without interjecting advice or condemnation. Allow them to vent their emotions. As they open up and display their frustrations or hostilities, check your knee-jerk reaction to correct. There will be time for that later.

Step Two. Maintain eye contact and give helpful responses, such as, "I see" or "Uh-huh." Even a simple nod of the head says, "I am listening and understand what you are saying."

Step Three. Reflect what you hear. In your own words, repeat what you just heard your youngster say. Try to pinpoint whether he is feeling angry, hurt, anxious, or excited. You may want to say something like, "It sounds like you are somewhat anxious about . . ."

With practice, these reflective statements will be second nature to you and will help you discern your child's emotional state.

When our kids are allowed to vent their hurts and frustrations, the intensity diminishes. Wouldn't you rather know your child is venting to *you* than to a less-than-desirable peer? As a parent, you are in a terrific position to be a channel for draining these powerful emotions. Also, kids are able to evaluate their feelings through venting. When they can verbalize their thoughts, hear how they sound, and then watch how others respond to what they say, they are better able to see the negative effects of their thoughts and behavior. Or, conversely, they may realize the thing they were so worried about is really nothing at all.

6. Thought Life

Enthusiasm and a positive approach to life will rub off on your kids. Modeling positive perspectives on life is the surest way to help your kids develop a healthy thought life. Many overweight kids are already depressed because of their criticism of themselves and others' criticism of them. A positive thought life greatly assists them in overcoming this negative outlook that soaks through to the inside.

Let your child know that even when situations are unpleasant and beyond our ability to change, we can change our view of it. We can either try to change the situation or accept it.

Following these six principles for ELICIT will help children feel good about themselves, as well as prepare them for the larger world of adulthood that awaits them.

Please don't walk away from this chapter feeling helpless or hopeless. As a parent, you hold a powerful key to positive, permanent change in your child's life. At the same time, realize that kids are cryptic. They won't typically come right up and tell you, "I feel lonely" or "I'm angry." Instead, you will need to learn how to read the signs they are sending. Once you gain their trust, you can ask the right questions—and always with sensitivity.

Key signs that a child is suffering in silence fall under the umbrella of exclusionary types of behavior: not being chosen for team sports or games; low confidence levels; always being alone; reluctance to join in a fun activity with a group of peers, such as a Friday night at the mall or going to see a movie where other kids will likely be.

Encourage him to talk to you about his feelings. If you suffered from obesity as a child, relate to him on that personal level and remind him of ways you overcame adversity or social rejection.

At the same time, remember that your child may have real struggles giving up their favorite foods. George Bernard Shaw once said, "There is no sincerer love than the love of food," and indeed, food is a part of life more primitive and fundamental than our most basic emotions. But, for many of us—including our children—food is so closely tied to emotions that it can quickly turn from a source of nourishment to something that causes harm.

The key to losing weight is to take control of the emotional challenges sabotaging your child's food choices. When you choose the right foods for your child, she will naturally lose weight and her body will function at its most optimum level; even her appearance will reflect this renewed level of health. There is no secret potion needed, only simple, basic foods and the commitment to stick with a new, healthier way of eating.

Of course, the hard part is not in understanding which foods to eat or avoid; the hard part is sticking to the program. Mentally, you and your child may know what the right foods to eat are, but emotionally you have been conditioned to crave certain foods, such as an abundance of grains and sugars. So in a very real sense, successful eating is not a battle of acquiring the right knowledge but a battle against emotions.

Hidden Feelings Behind Food Cravings

Perpetual fad dieting destabilizes a person's self-esteem and self-image. He briefly loses weight and then inevitably fails, returning to his previous, or an even heavier, weight. If your child has tried to lose weight in the past and failed, guess what that leads him to believe on a mental level? That he is an overweight person, and it's impossible for him to permanently lose weight. Further, on an emotional level, negative emotions or memories can prompt his taste buds to crave fattening grains and sugars to the point of addiction. The cycle is further encouraged on a metabolic level, where digestion and metabolism, overwhelmed by an excess of grains and sugars, tell his body to store fat.

It's important to break this cycle so that your child can return to a new home base—a home base where he is at his ideal, healthy weight. Breaking the cycle is where most people encounter problems, because behind food cravings lurk emotions that have to be dealt with before the cravings will subside.

Emotions are powerful. A person who is feeling sad, lonely, anxious, angry, or in need of comfort, compassion, or calm may be tempted to eat unhealthy foods as a way to cope with these feelings. The feelings are so intense, and the desire to deal with them by succumbing to food cravings is so strong, because behind those emotions are beliefs telling that person how to think, feel, and act, often without their realizing it. These are the emotional barriers your child needs to overcome.

Don't let negative emotions sabotage your child's efforts to feel good and reach her ideal weight. Food is an important part of life. On a practical side, look at your child's eating patterns. Determine to become involved as her partner in the quest for healthy living. It's been said there are two kinds of people in everyone's life: balcony people and basement people. Balcony people are the ones who cheer us on, shouting, "You can do it!" Basement people are those who discourage us and sink our confidence. As a parent, commit to become your child's primary balcony person, shouting encouragement every step of the way. Then, follow up that encouragement with the practical nutrition and exercise advice found in this book.

Baby Steps Lead to Success

Let's suppose for the sake of discussion that your child is eighty pounds overweight. The goal of losing that weight may seem insurmountable to both of you, but if you turn that gargantuan goal into a bite-size one, suddenly you and your child can track success.

The key for parents is to be helpful, not confrontational. For starters, you may simply encourage your child to eat more slowly or to cut back from three helpings to one at mealtimes. If your child eats more slowly, his brain will have time to register "full" before too much food is consumed. Now let's suppose you make this the goal for week one—or even month one. You've just created an easily attainable goal. There won't be a whole lot of physical change when you reach this goal, but you've made progress. Progress should be celebrated—but not with pizza and ice cream. Note your child's success in some way, such as on a progress-tracking board or by logging it in a journal.

Perhaps you decide to make maintenance the goal for now. You could approach this by saying, "Johnny, we both agree we want to reduce, and you have to understand that this is a long haul. I'll be here beside you the whole way, but for now let's just work on maintenance—let's not get any bigger." Psychologically, that is more helpful to a kid than saying, "Okay, Johnny, we've got to lose thirty pounds in the next three months, buddy."

A better approach would be to ask your child which physical activity she would most like to do. *Then help her do that activity!* If it requires your participation—whether through signing her up to a class/team or getting out and playing ball with her—just do it. Another option is to start a family activity program so the focus isn't trained entirely on "the kid with the weight problem." This can be as simple as an evening walk or bike ride around the neighborhood as a family. Your role-modeling is crucial.

Create a Parent-Child Contract

One effective means of enlisting your child's participation—and showing you're in this with him for the long haul—is to create a parent-child contract stating clearly what (attainable) goals and habits you want him to achieve. This could be a chart on the refrigerator or something you hang on the inside of your child's bedroom door. Make the steps/goals manageable so he can easily succeed and see progress.

For example, you might put in the contract a clause that says, "I will eat only one portion at dinner instead of three" and allow room for check marks each day of the week. Then, if he meets that goal for the week, reward him with a trip to the movies on Friday night or allow him one special "vacation food" (a favorite treat indulged in only occasionally—more on this in chapter 10). Or you might set a house rule that says TV and Nintendo time must be earned by doing forty-five minutes of physical activity every day. If you do make a contract with your child, however, be sure to follow through or they'll know you're only crying wolf.

Here's a sample contract:

Things I Will Do

Eat only one portion at every meal
Avoid junk food at school

Replace a bad dessert with a healthy alternative
Ride my bike for fifteen minutes after school
Go to soccer practice today

Suppose your child gets three out of five every day; that would be a great opportunity to reward him. Remember, however, that rewards don't really motivate; they're just rewards. The motivators have to be you, the parent; the contract; and the goal of looking and feeling better. Positive change is the best motivator of all, but knowing you are on his side will give a kid that extra fuel to go the distance with weight loss and learning new, healthy approaches to eating.

JUNK-FOOD NATION 3

The proper feeding of children is vitally important, as their bodies are literally being created by what they eat. Sadly, most American children eat (and are allowed to eat) food that can only safely be called junk food: refined foods and sugar-laden foods and beverages.

A steady diet of poor nutrition disrupts their health slowly over time, but sooner or later poor eating habits will take their revenge in the form of frequent illness, allergies, infections, adenoid problems, tonsillitis, weight gain, hyperactivity, learning disorders, and a host of other ailments. These symptoms of illness are signs that their young bodies are, quite frankly, being poisoned.

While children may burn up much of the excess sugars, chemicals, and additives found in these junk foods, ultimately they will pay the price for their unhealthy "kid diet." Have you ever found it strange that kids' menus in restaurants offer only a slew of fried meats, french fries, macaroni and cheese, or grilled-cheese sandwiches? Certainly no vegetables, healthy meats, or other nutritious foods—those are for the adults (if the adults choose to order them).

Children need healthy food perhaps more than anybody else does. Building their bodies out of a diet of junk food will not only affect their immediate health but will also limit their entire life potential. But, as everyone knows, junk food is so prevalent it's hard for many people (parents included) *not* to partake of this "quick-fix" diet. And that's no random coincidence. Consider the following.

How the Junk-Food Marketing Wizards Target Your Kids

As you pull into a vacant parking spot at the grocery store, you mentally tick off the few items you plan to buy. *This will be just a quick trip*, you promise yourself. But once inside, something changes the scenario—and your grocery list suddenly grows much longer. On the first aisle your youngster spots green gelatin pudding snacks. Hoping this one concession will make the rest of the trip easier, you cave in. But as you turn the corner into aisle two, your child starts begging for a bag of animal-shaped cookies.

By the time you leave the store you've racked up more than twenty dollars' worth of greasy, sugary, processed "foods" that may satiate your child's craving but will wreak havoc on his growing body.

It's no accident that kids crave these junk-food items. From the time they can sit in front of a TV screen and watch cartoons, children are exposed to the wonderful world of marketing. Over the years, junk-food marketers will target your child through TV, magazines, the radio, and even school, inundating them with the powerful messages of the junk-food industry.

According to the National Institute on Media and the Family, advertisements target children as young as three years old.[1] If adults find it hard to resist marketing ploys, imagine how difficult it is for a child to say no.

General Mills Inc., Kellogg Co., and Kraft Foods Inc.—the top three advertisers of packaged foods to children, by virtue of their breakfast cereals—now spend nearly $380 million a year on ads aimed at children in the U.S.[2] They know that children are persuasive "influencers" in every household, so if Johnny cries for purple Popsicles long enough, Mom or Dad will probably buy the product. The marketing ploys appear to be working, as one out of every four American children are now seriously overweight or at risk of becoming overweight.

Although the decision to purchase junk food lies with you, the parent, learning about the ways in which junk-food marketers target your kids can help you protect them from these unwholesome messages.

Athletes/Celebrities

Who of us isn't impressed by our favorite actor or sports celebrity? Many children view celebrities and athletes as role models. From there it's an easy leap to "buying into" the products they endorse. Children listen to the marketing messages because they like the messengers. Aside from the obvious message of "Buy this product" is the subliminal message that says eating this product can make them a celebrity or athlete—or at least look and perform like one.

Saturday-Morning Commercials

Saturday-morning cartoons are a long-standing tradition for American kids. You probably watched cartoons when you were a child. The big difference today, however, is how aggressive TV junk-food ads have become during those coveted few Saturday-morning hours. It is estimated that 90 percent of food commercials aired on Saturday-morning kids' TV shows are for empty-calorie products such as sugary cereals, candy, and fast food.[3]

Knowing the power of pop culture, junk-food marketers often feature a cartoon character or theme as part of their packaging and promotional angle. That's why, once you head to the grocery store, your child may light up at the sight of a certain cartoon-themed junk food. They've been "sold" that item many times over during the hours they watched the program, and now here it is right on the grocery-store shelf.

School Vending Machines

The days of hot meals complete with veggies are long gone from school cafeterias. Many parents are surprised to learn that their kids' school cafeteria resembles a fast-food court at the mall, complete with burgers, fries, and vending machines. Even if you send your child to school with a healthy lunch, your efforts may be sabotaged by junk-food marketers in a place that used to be a safe zone—your child's school. At a time when school hallways are lined with vending machines selling soft drinks and junk-food snacks, it's no wonder that so many kids are fat and getting fatter.

Indeed, junk-food and soft-drink marketers have invaded kids where they spend most of their time (the average student is in school seven hours a day). It's not uncommon for schools to make marketing deals with soft-drink companies such as Coca-Cola. As an incentive to carry the soft drink, schools receive commissions based on a percentage of sales, and sometimes even a lump-sum payment. While educators often use the revenues for academic and after-school activities, it's a poor trade-off for undermining students' health.

At the time of this writing, lawmakers and other policymakers are finally waking up to the epidemic of childhood obesity and the need to clean up our schools' food offerings.[4] Getting rid of vending machines in schools—or replacing their contents with pure water and healthy snacks—would make a huge difference in our children's health. Access to vending machines can increase consumption of soda by up to fifty or more cans per student per year.[5]

Fortunately, a growing number of states are striking back, trying to curb the rise in childhood obesity by placing strict limits on the sale of candy, soft drinks, and fatty snacks in schools. Nearly a dozen states are considering legislation to turn off school vending machines during class time, strip them of sweets, or impose new taxes on soft drinks to pay for teacher salaries and breakfast programs.

Many legislators are pushing to oust sodas from school machines altogether. Additionally, lawmakers are calling for a moratorium on soft-drink contracts that pay schools to dot their halls with soda machines.

The wave of legislation, unusual for both its breadth and its assertiveness, grew out of the newest statistics on child obesity from the Centers for Disease Control and Prevention. Teenagers today are almost three times as likely to be overweight as they were twenty years ago, the agency announced in 2005, prompting many lawmakers to take aim at the junk food they believe is to blame.

The Internet

Ever watchful for new marketing avenues, junk-food companies didn't take long to seize the realm of cyberspace. Many children have access to the Internet today, and Madison Avenue knows it. Little wonder, then, that every major junk food has its own promotional Web site, which typically caters to children and teenagers through interactive games featuring the product, giveaways, contests, and other information about the product.

Kids may be drawn in by the games, but once there they are inundated with images of the junk food or its brand. Although they may think they are simply playing a game, the power of subliminal marketing weaves its magic, sending the message that this is a "cool" product to eat or drink.

It's unrealistic to shield your children from all junk-food advertisements, but there are things you can do to limit the ads' influence. Sit down with your kids and explain that a business is selling the product; tell them they need to use their own common sense and not rely solely on the ads to make buying decisions. Make sure you are a good role model for your child. If you eat much junk food, you'll have a hard time convincing your kids they are better off avoiding it. Many people underestimate the power food can have on emotional health. Eating other junk foods or the wrong foods for your metabolic type will imbalance you not only on a physical level but also on an emotional one. This can easily leave you feeling irritable, nervous, angry, hyper, depressed, or hopeless. Similarly, the right foods will feed your body and your mind and will leave you feeling strong, energetic, in control, and emotionally sound.

In the struggle against obesity, the true enemy is not simply the processed foods themselves. Advertisers are diligently working day and night to come up with clever ways of tapping into the "junk-food junkie" that lives in many of us, tempting us daily to eat these "bad" foods. Their clever marketing ploys are working.

Just consider the following statistics from an ABC News July 27, 2004, report:

- McDonald's reportedly spent $500 million on one ad campaign while the National Cancer Institute spends about $1 million a year to promote eating five daily servings of fruits and vegetables.

- Junk-food advertisements target children as young as three years old.

- The food industry has a $30 billion advertising budget.[6]

You can stop being the target of these marketing strategies by making the decision to accept personal responsibility for your own health and what you eat. Realizing the cycle and being aware of the constant marketing of processed food around you—and educating your children about it—is a foundational initial step toward a healthier life. It's like the old saying "You are what you eat," and if that means mostly processed foods, you are setting yourself up for struggles with chronic degenerative diseases and far less energy and enthusiasm than you were designed to have. Surely you and your children deserve better.

Junk Food's Stranglehold

Someone once quipped that temptations would be easier to overcome if they weren't so tempting! Nothing could be truer when it comes to processed foods and their stranglehold on our cravings. Whatever your particular junk-food craving may be, you know it's not good for you—you may feel tired after you eat it, you may get a head rush or jittery feeling, and it might make you gain weight—but at the moment you want it.

What is it about processed food that makes us crave it, even though we know it really is what it claims to be—junk? Here are just a few of the reasons:

- Junk food tastes good.

- You use it to "reward" yourself.

- Your hectic schedule makes wholesome food preparation a chore.

- Processed foods make you feel good initially and may substitute for other areas in your life that are lacking pleasure (because of loneliness, depression, anxiety, stress, hopelessness, etc.).

- Convenience food is cheap.

You could probably add a few more points to the list yourself, but the conclusion remains the same: many people demand these nutritionally devoid foods. Now consider the following statistics:

- Americans spent $117 billion in obesity-related economic costs in 2003.[7]

- An estimated 300,000 Americans die each year from diet-related causes.[8]

- Food and beverage advertisers collectively spend $10–$12 billion a year to reach children and youth.[9]

- Americans now spend more money on fast food than on higher education, personal computers, computer software, or new cars.[10]

- Americans spend up to an estimated $50 billion a year on diet and weight loss.[11]

- Junk-food marketers spent an estimated $15 billion in 2002 solely on marketing aimed at children.[12]

Even though we pay lip service to wanting better nutrition options, it's clear from the above facts that the healthy-food message is no match for the processed food companies' advertising budgets. Maybe the ugly truth is that we are more susceptible to deceptive marketing than we are willing to admit. And if we find it hard to resist convenience foods as adults, just imagine what our kids must face. Unlike most adults today, children are being raised in a world where artificial foods are the norm and french fries constitute a "vegetable serving" (since, after all, french fries are made from potatoes).

Even more ridiculous is that popular diet books like *The South Beach Diet* promote french fries because they have more fat than potatoes and are less likely to cause weight gain, completely ignoring the serious dangers of trans fats.

Turning the Tide

Many new clients come to me complaining that whenever they try to eat healthily, they feel hungry and crave other foods. My response is always the same: you're probably not eating for your metabolic type, a nutritional philosophy built on the understanding that human bodies are unique and need to be fed according to their differing types. (We'll discuss metabolic typing in chapter 7.) If you eat the right ratio of proteins, fats, and carbohydrates—and the right types—for your metabolic type, you will naturally feel satisfied and full of energy. A wonderful side effect is that, when eating in this manner is combined with regular physical activity, your body will also rapidly and easily find and maintain your ideal weight.

Because the childhood-obesity epidemic has sounded a loud warning bell—and frightened many people—lawmakers are finally taking steps to reduce the prevalence of junk food in our society.

Fortunately, several initiatives are under way to help kids fight obesity on citywide, statewide, and sometimes even nationwide levels. One such example is PANA, the Pennsylvania Advocates for Nutrition and Activity. This statewide effort hopes to combat the epidemic of overweight and sedentary youth through participating schools, which commit to support healthy eating and physical activity as part of their total learning environment. More than nine hundred Pennsylvania schools have signed on since PANA's inauguration in February 2002.[13]

The first step in the right direction took place in 2001, when the U.S. surgeon general issued the "Call to Action to Prevent and Decrease Overweight and Obesity." That call to action essentially required the setting of agendas throughout the medical, educational, municipal, recreational, and commercial food-and-beverage sectors of American society. The problem, the U.S. surgeon general reasoned wisely, was not due to any one thing but an assortment of wrong lifestyle choices that combined to make an unhealthy whole.

In September 2004, the Institute of Medicine issued these recommendations for overcoming childhood obesity and creating more healthful lifestyles for American youth:

1. Parents—provide healthful foods, promote increased physical activity, and limit television and computer games.

2. Healthcare professionals—routinely track body mass index and provide needed counseling to children and their families.

3. Schools—develop new programs to teach about wellness, healthful eating, and exercise. Make sure school meals meet dietary guidelines and that all children participate in at least thirty minutes of physical activity daily. Conduct annual assessments of students' weight. Keep schools as advertising-free as possible.

4. Communities—provide programs for physical activities.

5. Fast-food and full-service restaurants—offer more healthy food and beverage options, including children's meals, and provide caloric content and general nutrition information.

6. Food and beverage industry—standardize serving sizes and develop packaging that emphasizes calorie content and nutrient density.

7. Recreation industry—offer increased options with regular physical activity.

8. Federal government—convene a conference to develop guidelines for the advertising and marketing of foods, beverages, and sedentary

entertainment addressed to youth. Give Federal Trade Commission authority to monitor compliance with guidelines.

9. Department of Health and Human Services—implement a long-term multimedia campaign aimed at prevention of obesity in children and youth.[14]

On a state level, organizations like PANA are leading the charge to bring back healthy, wholesome childhoods. Working through a vast network of leaders, volunteers, and concerned parents at every level of society, PANA has set aggressive but realistic goals for improvement, such as a 25 percent increase in participation in the Great Pennsylvania Workout Month (in 2004). Things like community-wide campaigns to provide healthy school lunches and the building of safe walking and biking routes are getting top priority in a system that might easily have ignored these issues in the past.[15]

On a personal level, PANA adherents commit to such behavioral changes as the following:

- Increase the number of adults who will participate in physical activities with their families.

- Limit television viewing to two hours or less per day for children and adolescents.

- Increase the proportion of children who walk to school within a distance of one mile or less.

- Increase the incidence of infant breast-feeding.

- Increase the number of adults who will commit to eat five servings of fruits and vegetables a day.

- Increase the proportion of parents who accept the use of BMI-for-age measure as a screening tool to assess growth patterns in children and youth.[16]

A similar initiative on the citywide level is the Consortium to Lower Obesity in Chicago Children, which has garnered collaboration across all sectors of society—including doctors, schools, museums, industry, and charity groups. Housed at Children's Hospital, CLOCC funds a variety of obesity-fighting projects and research throughout the city. The initiative has also become an information-sharing network that has amassed nearly seven hundred partners citywide.[17]

Meanwhile, with the success of its "Jared" Subway diet, the fast-food franchise known for being "fresh, not fried" has launched a School Lunch Program. Under the program, schools can either use contract delivery services or add on-site sandwich preparation to their cafeterias.

Subway also invites parents and kids to take its F.R.E.S.H. Steps Pledge (I Feel Responsible for my health and want to live my life Energized, Satisfied, and Happy). Those who sign the pledge promise to be more active, eat healthy foods, and create a healthy lifestyle. The franchise held a "March on Obesity" in Washington, D.C., on July 14, 2004, and Subwaykids.com provides an interactive forum for teaching kids the importance of being active and eating well.[18]

See Food, Want Food!

One recent government study showed how powerfully the sight of food impacts the brain's metabolism. When hungry people see or smell a favorite food, the study found, their brain reacts in a way similar to that of a drug addict upon seeing a drug. The regions of the brain that light up on brain scans when people are presented with a favorite food are the same areas that are associated with addiction. Put simply, this means that people have become junk-food addicts, and just the sight or smell of certain foods such as chocolate or pizza triggers a switch in the brain.

The study involved twelve people with normal and healthy body weights who were deprived of food before the study. The conclusions? The very sight of food significantly increased metabolism in the brain and resulted in hunger and desire for food. Not surprisingly, one researcher suggested that "advertising, candy machines, food shows, and food displays have kept our brains constantly in the 'on mode' whenever exposed to food stimuli thus greatly contributing to the obesity problem."[19]

Meanwhile, a second study showed how Americans have become complacent about their weight and have simply lost the will to do anything about it. In fact, many American physicians no longer advise their overweight patients to lose weight.[20]

So there are many hurdles to overcome—the junk-food advertisements, the perceptions about fat in America, even the way our brains react to food—and it's clear to see how we've become a junk-food nation—but fortunately there is a way out of this quagmire. In the following chapters you'll learn how to rescue your children from the processed-foods trap and set them on a healthy course for life.

HOW THE BODY GAINS —AND LOSES—FAT

4

Nothing motivates change like seeing results, so before we ask you to alter your child's food plan, let's explore the physiological reasons why such a radical change in your child's diet is necessary. Then, once you start seeing— and they start experiencing—positive results in their lives, you and your children will be strongly motivated to continue this new healthier way of eating.

An overwhelming number of studies over the past several years have confirmed that highly processed grains found in breads, pasta, cereals, potatoes, and rice, not fats, are what make you and your children fat. Even healthy grains like whole wheat, when refined and combined with refined sugars to make bread, can slow your metabolic function and promote weight gain, which leads to diabetes, heart disease, cancer, and strokes. Surprisingly, more than 90 percent of the population, even those at their ideal weight, seem to benefit from reducing their grain consumption.

Adopting a low-grain diet is an important step in keeping your child from transitioning from grain consumption to grain addiction. It's safe to say our nation is truly addicted to grains, and we are showing the side effects of this addiction in our collective weight gain and high levels of disease. If your child is overweight, and you don't aggressively address the problem, they will gain more weight and be on a collision course with insulin resistance that can lead to Metabolic Syndrome (formerly called Syndrome X), a precursor to diabetes. Some common symptoms of insulin resistance include high insulin levels, high blood pressure, elevated triglycerides, or low levels of HDL ("good") cholesterol. Insulin resistance is typically present but goes undetected for about a decade before type 2 diabetes is diagnosed.[1]

Many people find the above statements hard to believe. That is the way

I felt when I was in medical school. In fact, instead of *Joe,* my nickname in medical school was *Dr. Fiber.* I constantly lectured my classmates about the benefits of whole grains and how they could improve their health. I struggled for nearly twenty years before I finally learned enough to understand the science of how grain consumption is a primary factor contributing to the obesity epidemic.

While the fiber in whole grains can benefit your body's circulatory and digestive systems, there are other factors that have an overriding effect on your health. The vast majority of Americans struggle with insulin resistance. How do you know if you have insulin resistance? Well, nearly anyone with high blood pressure, type 2 diabetes, obesity, or high cholesterol has insulin resistance as a primary reason for their disease. Since two-thirds of Americans are overweight, once you factor in the other diseases, somewhere between 85 and 90 percent of people seem to benefit from avoiding grains, even whole unprocessed grains.[2]

While all grains trigger an insulin reaction, refined grains produce the most intense reaction because they are digested and absorbed much more quickly. These should be severely restricted in nearly everyone's diet. However, if you or your child has insulin resistance, it would be best to avoid all grains, even whole grains, until the symptoms of insulin resistance disappear, and then they can be gradually reintroduced.

How You Get Fat

Do you find it curious that after nearly two decades of touting "low-fat" as the cure for obesity, our nation is fatter than ever? Somewhere, our massive weight-loss experiment went horribly wrong. The truth is, while the nation's dietary recommendations focused our attention on reducing fat intake, the national consumption of grains, starches, and sweets skyrocketed, making us fatter than we were before.

Far from securing our weight-loss goals, this obsession with fat reduction proved disastrous. Why? Because typically the same person who eats "fat-free" bumps up their grain consumption to satisfy their hunger pangs—despite scientific evidence that starch-based diets promote weight gain, fat buildup, and higher concentrations of fat-producing enzymes. A leading source of calories used to be white bread, but in 2005, it shifted to sugar consumed in the form of sodas. The high-fructose corn syrup in sodas is made from corn, which is a grain.[3]

A large part of the responsibility can be placed on the recommendations of the government's food pyramid. Many are not aware that the scientists who developed these recommendations were not nutritionists but employees of the U.S. Department of Agriculture. There is ample evidence of a massive conflict of interest in the establishment of these guidelines. In my opinion, these guidelines benefited many corporate agriculture interests at the expense of the health of the U.S. public.

Fortunately, the USDA Food Pyramid guidelines, which previously urged us to consume six to eleven servings of grain per day, were revised in January 2005 to more healthful portions. The new guidelines suggest: "Eat at least 3 oz. of whole-grain cereals, breads, crackers, rice, or pasta every day."

Three Steps to Weight Gain

The simple truth is that successful weight loss is not just about limiting calories but rather controlling your insulin response. In this section you'll find out why. Many studies have confirmed that the key to successful weight loss is managing the carbohydrate-insulin-obesity connection. When your child drastically reduces her grain consumption, her body naturally reduces the production of insulin. So even though carbohydrates themselves are fat-free, your body stores these extra carbs as fat. This occurs in a three-step process, activated by the hormone insulin. Here's how it works:

Step One

When you eat carbohydrates, your blood-sugar level increases as the carbs are digested. Your body then releases insulin to lower the amount of sugar (glucose) circulating in your bloodstream. If you are a typical adult, you will have about one gallon of blood in your body. Most people don't realize that in all that blood there is only one teaspoon of sugar floating around. If the concentration went up to a tablespoon or two, you would go into a hyperglycemic coma and die.

Obviously your body has built-in protection mechanisms that prevent this from happening. If not for these mechanisms, you would die shortly after drinking a glass of orange juice, which may contain the equivalent of eight teaspoons of sugar.

The primary built-in protection your body has from preventing this problem is the production of insulin by your pancreas. The insulin your pancreas produces prevents you from dying in the short run. Unfortunately, elevated insulin levels will kill you in the long run through the accelerated development of chronic diseases like cancer, heart disease, and diabetes.

The calories have to go somewhere, and since your body has a limited capacity to store fuel as carbohydrates, insulin will help convert these carbohydrates into fat. Over time, the hormone insulin has evolved as the body's mechanism to store excess carbohydrate calories as fat in case of future famine. This is why insulin aggressively promotes the accumulation of body fat. When you eat a low-glycemic (blood-sugar-producing) food, such as a chicken breast or broccoli spear, blood glucose rises slowly. In this case, your body will release limited amounts of insulin and you will not have an excess of carbohydrates to be stored as fat.

Additionally, the insulin will also inhibit your body's ability to burn fat as a fuel. Consequently, anyone with elevated insulin levels will have enormous difficulties in losing weight, as the enzymes that cause you to burn fat are temporarily shut down or severely impaired by insulin levels.

Once this scenario starts, you are in trouble. The body will continue to gain more fat, and the fat perpetuates the problem and worsens insulin by releasing free fatty acids into the bloodstream. This in turn further worsens insulin resistance. It's a vicious cycle.

In addition to telling the body to store carbohydrates as fat, elevated insulin levels also send the message not to release any stored fat. After all, the body may need that fat for the upcoming "famine." This blocks you from using your stored body fat to produce energy. So the excess grains and sugars in your child's diet not only make him or her fat, but they also make your child *stay* fat. The insulin response must be moderated in order for the body to release stored fats and make them available to produce energy. The only way to do that is by avoiding or greatly reducing grains, starches, and sweets— all the high-glycemic foods.

Step Two

High insulin levels suppress glucagons and growth hormone. Glucagon plays a major role in maintaining normal concentrations of glucose in your blood and is often described as having the opposite effect of insulin—that is, it increases blood-sugar levels. Glucagon promotes the burning of fat and sugar in the body. Growth hormone is needed to increase the growth of muscle tissue. So a steady diet of grains, starches, and sugars signals your child's body to block the release of these two key fat-releasing hormones.

Step Three

Increased insulin levels cause hunger, perpetuating the cycle. After a meal with excessive grains, insulin rises in a struggle to lower your blood sugar. The result? You're soon hungry again. Perhaps you've noticed this trend in your children and wondered how they could be hungry so soon after eating. Now you know why. Typically, those cravings for sweets lead them to snack on still more grains and sweets. An attempt to ignore the hunger pangs through sheer willpower often leads to ravenous hunger and feeling shaky, moody, and like they're about to "crash." Once a person hits this stage, the body clings to that extra stored fat, and energy levels plummet.

Stated simply, this is called grain addiction. The grains and sugars your child is eating drive her to eat more of the wrong foods. This is the reason why most starchy vegetables, grains, and sugars can be addictive. Moderately reducing calorie intake from this food category, as some diets recommend, doesn't seem to work for most because the overweight person never breaks out of the cycle of insulin rise, fat storage, and cravings. Instead, the blood-sugar and insulin levels remain high, thwarting the body's ability to burn fat. As with any addiction, the only way to truly break free is to totally abstain from the addictive item—in this case sugar and grains.

For more-detailed information about the biochemistry of weight gain and weight loss, you may want to refer to my book *The Total Health Program* or search my Web site, www.mercola.com.

Beginner Nutritional Plan

Based on the simple biochemistry you've just learned about, the Beginner Nutritional Plan in chapter 6 will supply your child with foods that end the cycle of weight gain in the following ways:

1. By eliminating or greatly reducing the amount of grains, starches, and sugars consumed, you'll moderate the insulin response.

2. Increasing your child's intake of complex carbs from vegetables will stoke up his or her body's fat-burning capacity.

3. Eating foods like proteins and fats that don't produce an elevated insulin response will help your child feel nourished and full so he's not tempted to snack on the wrong foods.

4. By adding the right kinds of fats to their diet, you'll slow down carb digestion and absorption, helping to moderate the insulin reaction. On this eating plan, your child's hormone response will normalize and her blood-sugar, fat, and insulin levels will come back in balance—helping her to escape the obesity trap and its long-term health consequences.

The Beginner Nutritional Plan is composed of proteins, carbs, and fats. First, let's turn our attention to proteins, often referred to as the building blocks of the body.

Proteins: The Building Blocks of the Body

Humans need protein to live, period. Proteins have been called the body's "building blocks" because they are essential to the building, maintenance, and repair of body tissues such as your skin, internal organs, and muscle. They are also the major components of your immune system and most of your hormones. Proteins are made up of substances called amino acids—twenty-two of which are considered vital for health. You can make fourteen of these amino acids, but the other eight, known as essential amino acids, must be obtained from what you eat. Many types of foods contain protein, but only meat, eggs, cheese, and other foods from animal sources contain complete proteins providing the eight essential amino acids.

In my practice I've observed that many people don't eat enough protein. While protein intake varies from person to person and depends on your gender, height, weight, and exercise levels, a normal protein intake typically ranges from 20 to 50 grams per meal.

I've condensed my protein guidelines down to eight simple principles that will make the Beginner Nutrition Program easier to follow:

1. Your child can eat all meats in this phase. All meats, including lunchmeats, are allowed in the Beginner phase, although I would recommend purchasing lunchmeats that are preservative-free. The best type of meat, from a biological and an ecological perspective, would be from animals that are raised naturally. For chickens this would mean that they are free-range and not raised in a factory farm where they never see sunlight or eat insects. For beef, that would be grass-fed beef, as they avoid the industrial-type feedlots that most cattle go through where they are fed grains sprayed with pesticides, and they are injected with antibiotics and hormones to maximize their fat content.

2. Read the meat package label. If your child is eating packaged foods, read the label to find out the number of grams of protein per serving. For whole foods, 3 ounces of most meats will provide about 20 to 25 grams of protein. A 4-ounce hamburger, which is processed, has only about 20 grams of protein, while typical lunchmeats have about 5 grams per slice. One egg has about 6 grams of protein, and a cup of milk (not typically recommended) has 8 grams.

3. Eggs are actually healthy. Eggs have unfairly received a bad rap in years past, but they are an excellent source of protein. Here are a few guidelines for egg consumption:

- Go organic. Omega-3 eggs contain a 1:1 omega-6:3 ratio, while commercial eggs contain a 19:1 omega-6:3 ratio.

- Your child can easily eat one dozen eggs per week without causing a cholesterol increase. Scientists have shown that infants who eat the adult equivalent of forty eggs per week don't have any health problems.[4]

- Avoid artificial egg products, as they cost more and there is simply no need for them.

4. Restrict your child's intake of dairy products. Commercial pasteurized milk, yogurt, and cheese are allowed in the Beginner phase of the Total Health Program but are drastically reduced in the Intermediate phase. Raw-milk (unpasteurized) dairy products need not be restricted unless your child has a reaction to them. If your child has allergies, consider avoiding all dairy, or at the very least, milk. If your child likes yogurt, pay special attention to the carbohydrate content, as many contain added sweetener. Here's a surprise for you: low-fat dairy products are densely packed with carbohydrates and should be avoided.

5. Monitor your child's soy intake. Despite a lot of good press, most unfermented soy is really not that good for you. In the Beginner phase, however, all soy products are allowed. Among other issues, soy can weaken your immune system (input the term "soy" in the Mercola.com search engine to find dozens of articles on soy's health drawbacks). Soy products will be excluded in subsequent phases, with the exception of fermented soy products like tempeh, miso, and natto.

6. Watch your child's fish and seafood intake. Like soy, all fish and seafood products are allowed in this phase but are progressively eliminated in subsequent phases due to contamination with mercury and other toxins. Increasingly, most seafood and fish, regardless of their water source, have been shown to be consistently contaminated with mercury, dioxins, and PCBs. Most people think that farm-raised fish are an exception here, but they are actually worse. However, since children don't tend to be big fish eaters, this area may not be a problem for you.

7. Nuts and seeds are okay for now. Nuts and seeds are allowed in this phase but are progressively eliminated in subsequent phases. You may want to lower your child's nut intake now if any of the following conditions exist:

- Excess weight
- Obesity
- High cholesterol
- High blood pressure

Flaxseeds and walnuts are the only exceptions—both can be consumed in moderation in future phases, as they help your body balance omega-6 and omega-3 fats. (Most Americans consume dangerously low levels of omega-3 fats. Fish oil is the best source of omega-3 fats, as it contains the essential fatty acids DHA and EPA. Plant-based sources like flaxseed are among the next best choices, though they don't contain DHA and EPA.)

While it's true that seeds and nuts are relatively low in carbohydrates, nuts are dense sources of calories and should be used in moderation. You may want to wean your child off other nuts and allow her to consume only walnuts and flaxseed in moderate amounts.

Flaxseed: Several tablespoons of freshly ground flaxseed have plenty of water-soluble fiber, like Metamucil, and will help normalize bowel movements. It also tastes great.

Walnuts: Limit your child's intake of walnuts as they are dense forms of calories and could sabotage the weight-loss effort if more than a few per day are consumed.

Almonds: Should be limited. Many people use them because they feel they are a low-calorie snack. However, the high density of fat calories makes them very easy to overeat, so if consumed, please restrict them to about five or six per day.

8. Watch your child's bean and legume intake. For children who do not have a problem with insulin, beans and legumes are acceptable protein sources in this level. If your child does have high insulin levels, avoid feeding them beans until their insulin levels are stabilized. Once your child has achieved their ideal weight, you can introduce beans. As stated earlier, symptoms of high insulin levels include:

- Excess weight

- Obesity

- High cholesterol

- High blood pressure

Beans are sources of good, but not complete, proteins. Add some additional proteins to your child's meal if beans are their primary protein source for that meal. Also, be aware that beans contain carbohydrates.

Dispelling the Protein Myth

I often am asked whether *too much* protein consumption is bad for children and might cause ketosis. Popular diets like Atkins that allow unmoderated protein consumption can induce ketosis, a condition in which the body burns fat, producing a by-product called ketones. Ketosis is one of the body's last-ditch emergency responses when it has exhausted its carbohydrate stores. In varying degrees, ketosis can lead to muscle breakdown, nausea, dehydration, headaches, light-headedness, irritability, bad breath, and kidney problems. For all of these reasons I don't believe it is a wise or necessary way to lose weight. On the Total Health plan, your child will be eating abundant complex carbohydrates in the form of vegetables, which counteract ketosis by providing a source of carbohydrate fuel so their body won't need to burn fat exclusively for energy. This is a much safer and healthier way to lose weight.

Other questions I frequently hear: "Isn't it unhealthy to eat red meat? What if the red meat is not organic or grass-fed? Should I limit consumption?" Yes, commercial beef-raising practices are a genuine concern. To plump up their bodies—and subsequent sales in the market—cattle are given steroid hormones and antibiotics that transfer to the meat you eat. They are fed large amounts of pesticide-sprayed grain (primarily corn), which affects them the same way a grain diet affects humans—it "fattens" them up.

Grass-fed beef is preferable since, unlike commercial beef, it does not contain hormones, pesticides, or antibiotics. With beef, grass-fed is more important than organic as most grass-fed beef is essentially organic although it may not have official certification allowing the farmer to state that. But the bottom line is that if the cattle are not sent to feedlots and are given grains, that meets nearly all of the requirements of "organic" beef. Many farmers simply do not do the extra paperwork to obtain organic certification.

However, unless the cattle are grass-fed, their grain diet will transfer the negative insulin impacts to their human consumers. That's why I recommend grass-fed beef. The least expensive way to obtain this healthy protein is to find a local farmer who can sell it to you. This way you can avoid paying high shipping fees. If you are having problems finding it, for your convenience you can order direct from my Web site (www.mercola.com). Just type the key words "grass-fed beef" in the search engine at the top of any page on the Web site.

For most people, I do consider even nonorganic meats preferable to grains and sugars in the diet. However, there is a caution: elevated bodily stores of iron (resulting from eating red meat) can lead to heart disease and cancer. While children and menstruating women benefit from this extra iron, most adult men and non-menstruating women may have a problem with red meat consumption as it can raise their bodies' iron to unhealthy levels over time. This is easily monitored by checking the blood level of a protein called ferritin. You can use the search engine on my Web site for further details.

If you are concerned about food infections, it would be wise to cook ground beef until no pink remains, or until the meat temperature registers 160 degrees Fahrenheit. Slow-cooking methods that retain moisture work great on lean red meat. Braising is recommended for roasts, and low heat is ideal for steaks. Steaks should be cooked to a minimum of 140 degrees Fahrenheit (rare) and to a maximum of 160 degrees Fahrenheit (medium) to harvest the best tenderness and flavor.

By increasing foods like proteins and fats, which don't produce an elevated insulin response, your child will feel nourished and satiated—the best defense against the temptation to binge or otherwise indulge in the wrong foods.

Next we'll examine carbohydrates and why the right kind of carbs (complex) helps maintain a healthy, well-balanced body.

Carbohydrates: The Body's Power Source

Carbohydrates are your body's most efficient fuel source. Every time you fill up your car's tank with gas, you resupply its energy source. Your body is able to draw energy from two kinds of fuel sources (think of this as low- and high-octane). Carbohydrates provide fuel in the form of glucose, which is a sugar. What most people don't know, however, is that we don't actually need carbohydrates—they aren't essential for survival. If you ate no carbohydrates, just as many traditional Inuit (Eskimos) do, you would stay alive. Depending on your metabolic type, your health would increase or decrease on this type of diet.

There are two types of carbohydrates—simple and complex. Simple carbohydrates are sugars, such as the ones found in candy, fruits, and baked goods. Complex carbohydrates are starches found in beans, nuts, vegetables, and whole grains. From my perspective there is much confusion about complex carbohydrates. Technically speaking, unrefined whole grains are generally categorized as complex carbohydrates, and, as we explained earlier, even whole unprocessed grains can contribute to obesity.

I think it is easier to reclassify carbs into grain/sugar carbs and vegetable carbs. The carbohydrates typically found in vegetables are better for your body than those found in grains because the vegetable carbs have far more bonds for your body to break. This slows down the digestion process considerably and reduces the risk of raising your insulin levels. As mentioned earlier, grain carbohydrates actually increase insulin levels and interfere with your body's ability to burn fat.

Because grain consumption so directly affects insulin levels, I recommend that you scale back all grains, beans, and legumes from your overweight child's diet in the Beginner phase. The higher your child's insulin levels, the more ambitious your grain elimination should be. Grains to reduce include wheat, spelt, barley amaranth, millet, oats, rice, rye, quinoa, and teff. It is important to understand that though potatoes are actually a vegetable, the carb they contain is actually digested more like a grain—so please classify potatoes as grains. Additionally, many people believe that corn is a vegetable, but it is actually a grain.

The highly processed food products our culture has come to love are often the biggest culprits in generating increased insulin levels—and they should be the first to go. These include breads, pasta, cereal, bagels, french fries, chips, pretzels, waffles, pancakes, and baked goods.

Avoiding grains is a theme that I'll repeat often throughout this book, and I'll say it again here: for most of us, eliminating or greatly reducing grains is an essential strategy to successfully losing weight.

Not All Vegetables Are Created Equal

Vegetables are generally good, but some are much better than others. For example, increasing your child's vegetable intake with salads is a good start, but be sure to use dark leafy greens rather than iceberg lettuce. Why? Iceberg lettuce has minimal nutritional value. Red- and green-leaf lettuce, along with romaine lettuce and spinach, provide much more nutritious options. Once again, try to find organic vegetables, but if you're unable to obtain them, wash your nonorganic vegetables and remove peels and cores when possible.

My Recommended Vegetables list (provided in chapter 6) provides a guide to the most nutritious vegetables, as well as those to limit for their high carbohydrate content. A good rule of thumb: the greener and darker the vegetable, the more nutritious it will be. Finally, at least one-third of your child's diet should be raw foods, and vegetables are an obvious choice. Vegetable juicing provides an easy way to consume all the vegetables your child's body requires. You'll find several delicious juicing recipes in the recipe section of this book.

Curbing Your Child's Sweet Tooth

It's unrealistic to ask parents to put their child on a "cold turkey" diet of absolutely no sweeteners after years of sugar addiction. For that reason, the following sweeteners are acceptable during the Beginner phase of the program:

- Honey

- Rice syrup

- Beet sugar

- Maple syrup

- Molasses

Avoid using high-fructose corn syrup. Keep in mind, however, that the eventual goal is to wean your child off sugar in all its forms. Over time his taste buds will adjust and lose their craving for sweetness.

Your child may use artificial sweeteners at this level, but please avoid NutraSweet (aspartame), which is—in my opinion— by far the worst of the bunch. You can use acesulfame K and saccharin in moderation in this phase of the program. Using a sweetener increases sugar cravings in most people, so have your child use them with extreme caution. Please be sensitive to changes, such as an increase in sugar or grain cravings. If this occurs, you may want to stop the use of these sweeteners altogether.

Low-Carb Diets: Good or Bad?

Before we move on to the final macronutrient in the Total Health plan, fats, I feel it necessary to include a section about the low-carb craze that first became wildly popular in 2003. After an early spurt of enthusiasm when Dr. Robert C. Atkins introduced his diet philosophy in 1972, the Atkins Diet became the brunt of ridicule by scientists and doctors alike. Why? Because during the 1970s the prevailing dietary advice focused on a low-fat, low-calorie approach. As long as you avoided fats, your diet was considered healthy. But after three decades of Americans getting fatter on this low-fat advice, people started seeking other options that actually worked.

Dr. Atkins helped most Americans understand the importance of insulin and reducing the grains and sugars in their diet. By summer of 2003, more than two hundred low-carb specialty shops had opened across the nation.[5] The *New York Times* estimated that more than ten million people were following a low-carb diet regimen—and the food industry sat up and took notice, with everyone from food manufacturers to restaurant chains debuting low-carb products. TGI Friday's has partnered with Atkins Nutritionals to serve Atkins menu items at its five hundred–plus U.S. restaurants (the chain found that 19 percent of its customers are following the Atkins Diet). Meanwhile other restaurant chains such as P.F. Chang's China Bistro, Ruby Tuesday, KFC, and

Panera Breads have come out with their own low-carb entrée offerings. The sales of low-carb products exceeded $15 billion in 2003.[6]

There is no question the Atkins Diet has helped many people success-fully lose weight, but what is equally clear is that it has been a dismal failure for many others. Once you understand metabolic typing, the reason for these differing results becomes quite obvious. Surprisingly, about one-third of people actually need a high-carb diet to successfully lose weight. Of course, this would be a diet high in vegetable carbs; they still need to avoid grain and sugar carbohydrates.

1. One-third of the population requires a high-carb diet. Like so many failed dietary sanctions, the Atkins Diet offers a "one size fits all" diet. But, as we have already mentioned several times in this book, we are all unique. It is impossible to meet the diverse needs of the entire population with a one-size-fits-all dietary program. Any such program that claims it is good for everyone is bound to fail. Intuitively, most people know that what is healthy for one per-son may not be for another, and this perception is correct.

While most people lose some weight by following the Atkins program, the majority of them will eventually fail.[7] This is because these people actually require a higher-carb, lower-protein and fat diet, and the Atkins Diet does not provide the ideal fuel mixture they were genetically designed for. For these people, the Atkins Diet may even be dangerous, as the extra protein could cause kidney impairment if they already have some underlying problem prior to starting the diet.

2. Emotional factors are not addressed. Successful long-term weight loss and physical health are achieved in tandem with emotional health. No matter how hard you try to adhere to any dietary program, your child will not have success on it unless you first address her emotional factors. Anyone who's ever tried to lose weight knows that mastering this area is critical—you've con-quered the details, knowing what foods are "right" or "wrong," yet struggle nonetheless. The reason why is simple: our emotions wield a great deal of power over our rational minds.

Unfortunately, Dr. Atkins's program offers only temporary quick fixes to "emotional eating." But people caught in this emotional tailspin sorely need to address the underlying emotional factors that hinder their weight-loss efforts. In chapter 2, Dr. Em Twoey offers practical steps to help your child work through the emotional and psychosocial challenges children face.

Aside from the two major problems above, the Atkins Diet and other similar low-carb diets fall short in many other areas. Let's take a look at a few.

You Never Have to Count Carbs Again

Not only is counting carb grams a cumbersome and time-consuming way to live, it is also completely unnecessary. The Atkins Diet encourages the use of a "carbohydrate gram counter" to keep track of carb calories, especially during the Ongoing Weight Loss phase.

When your child eats according to their metabolic type on the Total Health plan, they eat until they are full and satisfied. Eating the ideal foods for your body negates the need for calorie counting, gram counting, or any other meticulous effort. Why? Because the body will naturally tell you when it's time to stop eating and when it's time to start.

Four final problems with the Atkins Diet are:

1. the recommended the use of sucralose, sold as Splenda®,

2. the encouraged consumption of nuts,

3. not enough emphasis on exercise, and

4. an underemphasis on food quality.

While nuts can have important health benefits, they are high in omega-6 fats. If you are not supplementing your child's diet with fish oils, their omega-6:3 ratio probably is closer to 15:1 rather than the ideal 1:1.

In my opinion, the Atkins Diet's recommended thirty minutes of daily cardiovascular exercise is simply not enough for weight loss. And in January 2005 the U.S. government echoed my advice by establishing its official recommendation of ninety minutes of daily exercise for those who need to lose weight. For most overweight people, twice that amount is needed. When you are trying to lose weight, this amount of daily exercise is necessary to increase the number of mitochondria in your muscles. Doing so increases your body's metabolic rate so that it continues to burn calories at rest and even while sleeping.

For children, getting one hour of exercise may be easier than it sounds—certainly easier than it is for the average sedentary adult. Middle schoolers and high schoolers rack up half an hour of quick-paced walking getting from one classroom to another throughout the course of a school day on a large campus.

(Usually they have only five minutes to do so for each class period—that's hustling!) Depending on their age, encourage your child to get another half hour of exercise by doing lawn chores, playing outside, walking to and from school (within a reasonable distance), engaging in team sports, or any of the other suggested exercise options mentioned in chapter 11.

Finally, the quality of the food your child eats is extremely important—something the Atkins Diet does not stress. A diet of factory-farmed animals and pasteurized dairy will expose them to toxins and nutrients devoid of their beneficial qualities. Though little emphasis is placed on food quality in the diet industry, it is just as important as the type of food being eaten. Unfortunately, the Atkins Diet gained a reputation for allowing less-than-ideal foods such as processed meats and processed low-carb energy bars. There are three major areas that need serious revision:

Beef: Whenever possible, choose free-range grass-fed cattle rather than cattle-fed grains. When you eat grain-fed beef, the fat composition actually changes and becomes unfavorable for health. Grass-fed beef, on the other hand, is highly health promoting, provided it is right for your metabolic type.

Milk: Dr. Atkins endorses liberal amounts of dairy in his program, but many people suffer significant complications from consuming commercial pasteurized dairy. Problems range from lactose intolerance to far more serious health complications. The good news is that choosing raw dairy—as opposed to pasteurized—will eliminate these risks.

Fish: For decades fish has been touted as one of the healthiest foods you can eat, and both the Atkins Diet and the South Beach Diet recommend hearty amounts in your diet. Sadly, the fish and seafood available today are likely to contain mercury and PCBs, regardless of their original water source. Generations of water pollution from coal plants and other factories have contaminated our freshwater supplies, which then flow into the ocean. Mercury and PCBs can lead to all kinds of very serious disease, including neurological disorders.

Many health practitioners and major health and government agencies (including the EPA and the FDA) have warned against the dangerous levels of these toxins in seafood and fish. One safe way to obtain the health benefits of omega-3 fats, yet avoid the mercury and PCBs in fish, is to substitute high-quality sources of fish or krill oil in a liquid or capsule form.

So while Dr. Atkins deserves praise for his groundbreaking work, some refinements are required to take it to the next level. It is this next level that will help people achieve the high level of wellness they are seeking, and no one understood better than Dr. Atkins that such well-intentioned criticism—insight offered to truly help people—is precisely what drives real progress in health care and medicine.

So how do you know if your child needs a low-carb or a high-carb diet? The condensed version of the metabolic type test in the next chapter will supply the answer. (If your child is very young, do your best to discern the correct answers from their eating patterns.) Understanding your child's metabolic type will equip you to know what next steps to take with this critical knowledge. The test requires some number crunching, so if you would rather have the computer do it for you, please go to my Web site (www.mercola.com) and type in "metabolic typing" on the search engine. You can take the free short form of the test.

FIRST LOW-CARB BOOK NEARLY 150 YEARS OLD

If you thought the low-carb revolution got its start with Dr. Robert C. Atkins in the 1970s, think again. It turns out a British undertaker named William Banting beat Atkins to the publishing market by more than a century—with surprisingly similar dietary advice.

Banting's low-carb diet theory started with a small booklet titled *Letter on Corpulence Addressed to the Public*. First published in 1863, the booklet went into many editions and stayed in publication long after the author's death.

Suffering from obesity, numerous health problems, and disturbed sleep, Banting came into contact with a doctor who challenged him to try a new way of eating. Dr. William Harvey's basic advice was for Banting to give up bread, butter, milk, sugar, beer, and potatoes, all of which contained starch and saccharine (sugar). On his new diet Banting was allowed:

- up to six ounces of bacon, beef, mutton, venison, kidneys, fish, or any form of poultry or game;

- the "fruit of any pudding"—but not the pastry;

- any vegetable except potatoes;

- at dinner, two or three glasses of claret, sherry, or Madeira;
- tea without milk or sugar; and
- only one ounce of toast.

Within a few days, Banting was sleeping soundly for six to eight hours per night, and his other health problems gradually waned. The undertaker dropped nearly one pound per week over the course of a year, losing forty-six pounds of weight and twelve inches off his waist. In his booklet, Banting would later write with enthusiasm, "I can confidently state that quantity of diet may safely be left to the natural appetite; and that it is quality only which is essential to abate and cure corpulence."[8]

Feed Your Head—with Fats

Here's a fun fact many people don't know: the human brain is made up of about 60 percent fat. It goes without saying, therefore, that fats are a very important part of your child's diet. The fats we eat strongly influence our level of brain function, and some nutritional anthropologists believe the human brain's development is due to our distant ancestors' access to high levels of DHA (a type of fat) found in fish and wild game. After only two generations of high omega-6 and low omega-3 fats, humans show profound changes in brain size and function.

Fat is composed of fatty acids attached to a substance called glycerol. The importance of fat's role in the body cannot be overstated; fats are essential to build cell membranes, clot blood, absorb vitamins, cushion vital organs, and protect us from extreme temperatures.

Following are a list of guidelines to keep in mind as you start your child on the Total Health plan:

1. The Type of Fat Matters, Not the Amount

Perhaps no other macronutrient has generated such conflicting information as fat. No wonder people are so confused about fats. When you go to the grocery store, you're confronted with advertisements claiming a product is low in fat or made with partially hydrogenated oil. To make sense of all the labels, I've compiled the following list of definitions:

Saturated fats: Found in animal products such as butter, cheese, whole milk, ice cream, cream, and fatty meats, saturated fats are also found in some vegetable oils—namely coconut, palm, and palm kernel. Saturated fats are not as dangerous as you have been led to believe. The demonization of fat has a long story that is beyond the scope of this book.

Most people don't realize that about one-third of their brain is saturated fat. Coconut oil has been an unfortunate victim of the pervasive saturated-fat myth. It is actually quite healthy and my recommended oil for cooking since it is far less likely to be damaged through frying. Coconut oil also contains a fat called lauric acid that some experts believe may even be an essential fat.

Trans-fatty acids: These fats form when vegetable oil hardens, a process called hydrogenation, and can raise LDL (bad cholesterol) levels. They can also lower HDL (good cholesterol) levels. Considered very dangerous, these fatty acids have been linked to heart disease. Avoid them in your child's diet (and your own). Fortunately, the FDA has mandated that all food manufacturers include them on the package label.

Monounsaturated fats: The best oil in the monounsaturated category is olive oil, which I strongly prefer over canola oil. Olive oil has a history of thousands of years of being used as a health food, while canola oil is relatively recent, and many experts are concerned about some of its properties.

2. Omega-3 and Omega-6 Fats Are a Dietary Must

Other than increasing the intake of water and fresh green vegetables, consuming fish oil is my strongest dietary recommendation to prevent disease and live longer.

Americans' intake of omega-6, a fat found in corn, soy, sunflower, and other oils, is far too high, while we simultaneously consume a dangerously low amount of omega-3 fats. Found only in fish oil and some plants, omega-3 fats are essential to good health. The ideal ratio of omega-6 to omega-3 is 1:1, but the typical American's ratio ranges from 15:1 to 50:1. To state it simply: for every omega-6 fat our distant ancestors ate, they ate one omega-3 fat; most Americans consume fifteen omega-6 fats for each omega-3 fat they eat!

Although omega-6 fats are considered an "essential" fat, in Western cultures it is extraordinarily difficult to ever become deficient in them. At the end of the nineteenth century Americans consumed very little vegetable oil, which is primarily omega-fat. By the end of the twentieth century, consumption had increased to seventy-five pounds per year of highly processed vegetable oils. I believe that with the exception of gamma linolenic acid (GLA) for some, omega-6 supplements are a complete waste of your money and should be avoided.

This lack of omega-3 fats in our diets may be a primary reason for the diseases Americans face, as well as our shorter life spans compared to many "first-world" countries such as Japan or Greece.

Benefits of omega-3 found in fish and krill oil include the following:

- Increased energy level and ability to concentrate

- Greater resistance to common illnesses such as flu and cold

- Prevention of heart disease, cancer, depression, Alzheimer's, arthritis, diabetes, hyperactivity, and many other diseases

Omega-3 fats DHA and EPA are essential for brain and nerve function. Omega-3s improve your cells' response to insulin, neurotransmitters, and other messengers. When your cells are damaged, omega-3 fats help in the repair process. Omega-6 fats, on the other hand, contribute to insulin resistance, alter your mood, and impair learning and cellular repair. You can see why avoiding high levels of omega-6 fats is important. To do so, have your child avoid all vegetable seed oils.

Striking a balance is key when it comes to omega-3 and omega-6 fats. On the Total Health Program, you will have to consciously feed your child omega-3 fats while lowering their omega-6 fat intake. Failure to lower omega-6 fats to acceptable levels will result in an unacceptable omega-6:3 ratio, and your child will not receive many of the wonderful benefits of omega-3 fats. The benefits that you will notice most in your children are these:

- Increased intelligence

- Decrease in any ADHD behavior

- Decrease in allergies and asthma

- Decrease in occurrence of colds, coughs, and flu

Flaxseed, chia seeds, walnuts, and a few other foods contain omega-3 fats, but the most beneficial form of omega-3 is found in fish because fish also contains the longer chain omega-3 fats, DHA and EPA, which are far more important in the prevention of both physical and mental disease. Plant sources like flaxseed, while helpful to consume, do only have the shorter chain omega-3 fat ALA; only a tiny percentage is converted to the beneficial EPA and DHA fats that are found in fish and krill oils. However, as I've stated before, your child will be better off consuming fish oil and krill oil rather than actual fish because of the contaminants in our water sources.

3. Be Sure Your Child Consumes Fish Oil in the Right Amounts

Let your child take fish oil in the warmer months and cod-liver oil in the fall, winter, and early spring months. Although this recommendation may sound strange, there's a solid reason behind my recommendation: cod-liver oil is high in vitamin D, and your child's vitamin D levels are often too low in cool months but adequate in warm months (the sun is a primary source of vitamin D). If you live in the southern states, this might be only two to three months of the year, but for those in the cloudy northern states that time could be as long as four to six months.

Most people can safely take up to one teaspoon of cod-liver oil for every twenty-five to forty pounds of body weight during the winter, early spring, and late fall months. Just be sure you don't neglect this very important fat—omega-3 fat deficiencies have been tied to the following problems:

Lack of mental sharpness on awakening	Lack of quality sleep	Depression
	Weight gain	Dry hair
Memory problems	Dry skin	Allergies
Brittle fingernails	Arthritis	Fatigue
Inability to concentrate		

The normal dose of fish or cod-liver oil for your child is one 1,000-mg capsule with 300 mg of EPA/DHA for every ten pounds of body weight. This dosing works well up to 150 pounds of body weight. Ideally, the dose should be divided equally over three meals. One teaspoon of fish or cod-liver oil is equal to about five capsules, and there are three teaspoons in one tablespoon, so one tablespoon would equal about fifteen capsules of most fish or cod-liver oils.

Krill oil requires much less because it has increased absorption due to its phospholipid component. So the typical adult dose is two 500-mg capsules per day. One of the benefits of using krill is that it is from the largest biomass in the ocean, so there is no concern about depleting the world's supply of this valuable source of omega-3 fats. Additionally, because they grow to only one inch long and are typically harvested from the Antarctic Ocean, they are virtually free of toxins and require very little processing to clean them up. One additional benefit is that krill do not cause the belching or burping that plague many when they consume typical fish oil products.

After you start the fish or krill oil, watch your child to see whether one or more of the symptoms of omega-3 fat deficiencies improve. If after a time on the fish oil your child's symptoms return for no apparent reason, he is probably taking too much fish oil. Stop his dose for a short while to help his body eliminate the oil and then resume at a lower dose.

Following the above guidelines will help fine-tune your child's dose to a fully beneficial level of omega-3s.

In the next chapter we'll explore the foundational element of creating a healthy diet—learning your child's metabolic type. Once that factor is in place, you will be equipped to help your child find her way into the health and fitness zone and into a place of sustained health and optimal weight.

THE HEALTH AND FITNESS ZONE

5

Built into the matrix of popular diets is the guarantee of failure. Fad diets may work for a while, and you may see eager dieters drop several pounds fast, but check back with those same people one year later and most will have gained back all the weight—and then some. Have you ever wondered why ads for popular diets contain the fine-print disclaimer "results not typical"? Well, now you know. Going on a fad diet is one of the worst things you, or your child, could do to your body. That's a blunt statement, but I can say it with all authority, backed by more than twenty years of research and real-world experiences from the tens of thousands of patients who have walked through the doors of my Optimal Wellness Center in the Chicago area.

Since you're reading this book, you may already have an overweight child, or you may want to set your son or daughter on the path to a lifetime of health, and that includes reaching an ideal weight he or she can easily and permanently maintain. You deserve the truth about healthy weight loss and a program that guarantees "results are typical" for a change.

Since you're seeking real, workable solutions to transform your child back to health and fitness, the last thing you need is one more miraculous-sounding promise. Every day we're bombarded by far-fetched claims for new diets, supplements, pills, and programs promising easy, permanent weight loss, but delivering disappointment instead. Enough is enough. Along with Dr. Lerner, I'm going to show you how the eating and exercise precepts in this book will truly improve your child's health, weight, and quality of life.

The recommendations contained within these pages are the result of more than twenty years of dietary and clinical research. Back in the late 1970s, when I was still in medical school, something kept telling me that eating a proper diet was the key to health and healing, even though the focus of the medical world was almost entirely trained on cures rather than prevention. A few years later, as a young physician I began working in the area that would become my life's mission: to discover through committed investigation the ideal diet to help people prevent chronic disease and weight gain and to reach their highest potential.

From the late 1980s through the early 1990s, my perception of the conventional healthcare system underwent a profound shift—I realized that its foundation is fatally flawed, centered on treatments and band-aid remedies rather than prevention. The system also seemed to disregard the healing powers that God built into each and every human body. As I looked around I saw that people were genuinely confused about what the "right" diet consisted of— and understandably so.

The fad diets gave conflicting advice about how much protein, fats, and carbs to eat. Meanwhile, the fast-food industry led people toward horrible food choices, and the pharmaceutical industry—fueled by the billions of dollars it stood to gain—encouraged Americans to pop a pill for everything that vexed them. People deserved the real answer, not information tainted by politics or greed, and I was committed to finding that answer.

Over the years I've been asked what are the main dietary and lifestyle changes a person can make to improve their health most dramatically. Here are the big four:

1. Most people would benefit from radically changing the types of fat they are eating. They need to:

    - Reduce the amount of omega-6 vegetable oils

    - Increase the amount of high-quality fish or krill oil omega-3 fats in their diet

    - Decrease, or ideally eliminate, trans fat in their diet

    - Use healthier, more stable, fats, like coconut oil for cooking

    - Use high-quality olive oils

2. Vastly reduce the amount of grains and sugars you and your child consume. It is primarily your body's response to the overindulgence of grains and sugars, not the intake of fat, that makes you fat.

3. Recognize that emotional health is directly related to physical health. Your child needs to know that you are his or her champion in the quest for wellness and a healthy weight. Your encouragement and participation in the process will greatly improve his or her ability to go the distance.

4. Learn how to identify your child's metabolic type. We all have a unique biochemistry, or metabolic type, and there are specific foods, at specific portions or levels, that are most ideal for each type. Conversely, some foods that are generally considered "healthy" may not be as healthy as you were led to believe. One of the important keys to finding and maintaining your ideal weight is learning the major metabolic typing principles for dietary success. In chapter 7 you'll learn how to assess your child's metabolic type and how to shape a food plan that fits her body's unique needs. But first let's take a look at some basic human physiology so you can begin to understand why grains and sugars especially should be avoided.

From Hunter-Gatherers to Grain Junkies

Your body wasn't made to consume a diet of grains, sweets, and starchy foods. In order to find out why, we need to dig into the past, back to the time of our ancestors. For more than five hundred generations, our distant ancestors existed primarily on a diet of wild animals and vegetation. They literally lived off what they hunted and gathered. But when society changed from hunting-gathering to agriculture six thousand years ago, humans began eating large amounts of sugar and starch in the form of grains and potatoes. Since nearly all our genes were set before the advent of agriculture, in biological terms our bodies are still those of hunter-gatherers.

History paints this as a beneficial change for mankind, but a growing body of evidence suggests it may have had negative health repercussions. Consider the lifestyle of the ancient Egyptians. With plenty of fruits, vegetables, stone-ground whole wheat bread, occasional meat, and olive, safflower, flaxseed, and sesame oils, the Egyptians' diet seems nutritionally sound. Yet when studies compared thousands of Egyptian mummies to the remains of hunter-gatherer societies, they found the following:

- Hunter-gatherers lived longer.

- Agriculturists had more infections and tooth decay.

- Heart disease and arteriosclerosis were more prevalent in mummies.

- Obesity, particularly abdominal obesity, was common among the Egyptians.[1]

Nutritional anthropologists found evidence in fossil records and other sources supporting the hypothesis that our bodies are genetically designed to fare better on the hunter-gatherer's diet—or a diet closer to it. According to their research, widespread grain consumption had the following negative consequences:

- Decrease in height

- Increase in infant mortality

- Decrease in life span

- Increase in infectious diseases

- Increase in dental disease and tooth decay

- Increase in bone diseases like osteoporosis[2]

The grains consumed in ancient times were 100 percent organic and unrefined, yet still had these negative health impacts. Today, 90 percent of our grains are highly processed, only making matters worse. Several studies of historical eating patterns show that our current level of refined carbohydrate consumption is unprecedented. Are our bodies designed to process the volume of grain and sugar carbohydrates with which we bombard them in modern diets? Clearly, the answer is no—and here's why.

Glucose Overload

One of the most serious health problems caused by grain consumption is elevated blood-sugar levels, which trigger cravings for sweets, and elevated insulin levels—the chief culprit behind many health problems. Americans consume dangerous quantities of sweets. Before 1900 sugar was a luxury item, saved for special holidays and rare occasions. In the last one hundred years, sugar (and sweetener) use has doubled.

According to the U.S. Department of Agriculture (USDA), between 1970 and 1993 the annual consumption of corn sugar alone increased from nineteen pounds to seventy-nine pounds per person. For the last decade, overall sugar consumption rose nearly 1.7 percent a year. In 2004, the average American consumed a whopping 175-plus pounds of sugar, 20 percent of it in soda. And along with this expanding consumption our waistlines have grown proportionately! This is the horrific legacy we are leaving our children.

Diet Disasters

At the beginning of this chapter I told you that fad diets are practically guaranteed to fail. The reason why is simple: most diets fail due to cravings for grains and sugars, which are symptomatic of grain addiction. Let's face it—no one's addicted to spinach or other healthy greens, which contain complex carbohydrates. But many people fall off the diet wagon reaching for breads, pasta, pizza, ice cream, or cookies. The best-selling book *The Carbohydrate Addict's Diet* first drew national attention to the prevalence of carb addiction and its subsequent health dangers. But despite its astute diagnosis, which rang true for millions of readers, Drs. Heller and Heller's food plan proved ineffective for many people. Why? Because it allowed dieters to eat ample quantities of grains, starchy foods, and sweets for a brief period every day.

Reprogramming the Body

Diets fail because after the "diet" you return to your old eating habits. It's not because you're weak-willed; it's because you do what your body *tells* you to do. Even the most disciplined person can stick to a strict deprivation diet for only so long. For children, a deprivation diet is even more unfeasible—and disastrous. And most diets are just that—meant for a short time period because they are too restrictive either in nutrients or satiety for anyone to follow in the long run.

More than 175 million Americans are classified as overweight (with a staggering 80 million of these classified as obese). Why? Because they did what their cells told them to do—they kept eating grains and sugars. With a new way of eating and new wiring, however, anyone can erase the old tapes and create a biological response that works in their favor. I call this *reprogramming the body*.

When I first began my practice as a physician, I watched helplessly as patient after patient got caught in the cycle of diet followed by weight gain. The frustrating cycle left them discouraged, ready to throw up their hands and give in to the notion that they were simply "designed" to be fat. In 1995, I was fortunate enough to attend a lecture on insulin physiology by one of the top experts in the country on this topic, Dr. Ron Rosedale, who authored *The Rosedale Diet*. His three-hour lecture convinced me that insulin was the cornerstone to optimizing weight loss and preventing nearly all chronic degenerative diseases.

I immediately incorporated this plan into my practice and observed an explosion in the success rate of the majority of the people who adopted it. However, it clearly did not work for everyone, as many people simply did not respond well to the high-protein diets I was advising them to follow. Little did I know at the time that these "carb" types actually required a very low-protein, low-fat, and much higher-vegetable diet. It wasn't until seven years later when I learned and applied the principles of metabolic typing that I found a diet that worked for nearly everyone. Interestingly, metabolic typing also explained my confusion as to why some people (carb types) responded so well to fresh green vegetable juice, and others (protein types) did not do nearly as well on this miracle superfood.

This is the only dietary program I am convinced is designed to benefit well over 95 percent of the people who use it. No other program even comes close. After twenty years of diligently searching for the truth of what is the ideal diet, I was finally able to learn the foundational universal principles that would benefit nearly everyone who applied them.

The cornerstone of this program (which is outlined in detail in my book *Total Health Program*) is one simple secret to effortless weight loss: eliminating or greatly reducing from your diet the following:

- Grains

- Starches

- Sweets

Total elimination of these food groups is the ideal for a child who is overweight (adding back small amounts of whole grains once his or her weight is stabilized), but even if you drastically reduce consumption of these foods, your child will lose body fat and gain significant health benefits. With this eating plan, you're going to get serious about weight loss for your child and take a giant leap forward. For a certain time period, you will restrict grains and sugars in order to change the messages his body sends him.

My weight-loss strategy constitutes a total reprogramming of the system for permanent weight loss. Total systemic reprogramming will transform your child from a kid who struggles to be happy with her weight to a slim child in control of food addictions and cravings—forever.

Here's how it works:

1. Once you start eliminating the recommended foods from your child's diet, his or her cells get this new message: release fat and burn it. The end result: weight loss.

2. Emotions can play a powerful role in food cravings as well as overeating. On the Total Health Program, your child's cells will send her the message to eat nutrient-rich foods instead of telegraphing the urge to eat fattening foods. The end result: your child will conquer food cravings and overcome grain and sugar addictions.

A steady diet of the right foods, coupled with positive affirmations and the other emotional health tools found in this book, will lead to a healthy body and improved self-image.

Starting Young

It goes without saying that you should start your children, from infancy, on the right food. We were all designed to be breast-fed, so every effort possible to implement this food for the first year of life will reap tremendous health benefits for your child. After she is off breast milk, offering your child the correct foods is the single most important nutritional gift you can give her. Once your child has reached the age of six years, you have lost your most significant opportunity for influencing major changes; so the younger you start, the better off your child will be. Many parents feed their children junk food because "they won't eat anything else." While it can certainly be a struggle to get children to eat healthy foods, especially if they are older and accustomed to less-than-ideal eating habits, simply offering only healthy foods to your children is what's best for them.

I have implemented this strategy for many hundreds of children and can assure you your child will not starve. Children are born with a reflex that will automatically trigger their appetite for nearly any food once their calorie intake dramatically decreases. The only time this mechanism does not kick in is when there is a profound brain injury. So unless your child falls in this category, you can rest assured that restricting their food selections to healthy foods will nearly always rapidly result in their adopting the new foods.

If she won't eat the foods you're offering, don't allow her to eat junk food instead. Sooner or later, your child will eat the healthy foods you've offered. And once she realizes how much healthier she feels, she's likely to start choosing them on her own shortly thereafter. Remember to always implement the changes in love—and *never* force your child to eat anything.

In the next chapter we'll take a look at the cornerstone of my health practice, the Total Health Beginner Nutrition Plan, and examine four time-tested gauges of health that you can use to determine your own child's level of health.

THE RIGHT FOODS: HIGH-OCTANE FUEL FOR YOUR CHILD

6

Whether your child is struggling with weight issues, facing a disease or condition, or you consider them reasonably healthy, the recommendations summarized below will help him achieve the healthy life he so richly deserves.

So what makes the Total Health Program different from all the other diets you've tried? It's based on hard scientific data and tried-and-true principles. There are no miracle cures here, just tools to help you understand your child's body and achieve optimum health. For too long now, leading dietary experts have promoted one-size-fits-all solutions to the nation's obesity problem, but that thinking is intrinsically flawed. If it were not, few of us would be overweight. Since the opposite is true, we can conclude that something is very wrong with the shotgun approach to nutrition. Although certain universal truths exist, such as the dangers of sugar and toxins, my experience in working with tens of thousands of patients has taught me that each person needs a custom fit.

Fact: What's good for one person may be toxic to another.

Due to differences in metabolic biochemistry, many diets will reverse a condition in one person but have no effect, or even worsen the condition, in another. Our biochemical and physiological "fingerprints" are unique, just as we differ from other people in the way we look physically. It should come as no surprise, then, that each of us processes foods and uses nutrients differently. When you adopt a diet based on your child's specific metabolic type, you help your child achieve optimum health.

Addressing health from your metabolic-type standpoint has a powerful end result: your health problems are treated at the foundational level, producing a permanent solution for regaining your health rather than treating symptoms, which only provides temporary relief.

Before we examine the nutrition plan in-depth, let me assure you of two very important facts:

1. Your child will not have hunger pangs. You can put your fears to rest. When you feed your child according to their specific nutritional requirements, she will not have any hunger pangs. This is because balancing the diet needs makes food cravings disappear. On top of that, your child will wake up each day full of abundant energy. Conversely, if she has "too much" energy during the day, as many ADHD children appear to have, she will actually calm down and be able to focus and concentrate and finally carefully listen and follow instructions. If this isn't happening, consider it a giant clue that you are not giving her body something it needs, and you will have to modify her program.

2. You can do it! It can be difficult to overturn years of improper eating patterns, but remember: this eating program is manageable for a reason—so you and your child can succeed! Start your child on these healthy eating recommendations with a just-do-it attitude, and you'll soon find your own built-in set of motivators in the form of gradual fat loss for your child and optimized wellness.

Jump-Start the Program

The Total Health complete nutrition plan is broken down into three phases: Beginner, Intermediate, and Advanced. We already talked a little about this in chapter 4, but we'll get into more specifics here. Those who are already implementing my nutritional advice are exceptions to this rule, but to keep things simple we'll focus on the Beginner phase here, where almost everyone should begin—especially children. Those with serious diseases or other conditions may want to take the more-extensive advice found in all three stages to promote healing and health.

My reasons for starting at the Beginner level are twofold:

1. The basic requirements in this level will take time and patience to integrate into your child's daily eating patterns.

2. Your child's body will need time to adjust to lowered insulin levels.

Before starting the program, it's critical to assess your child's "Four Factors"—insulin, weight, blood pressure, and cholesterol—as defined in the next few pages. Doing so will help you determine which areas to put the most initial focus on. From time to time be sure to monitor these four factors as a means of tracking your child's progress through the program. Fluctuations in the wrong direction will provide a crucial key that you need to make adjustments in the plan.

Some of the changes you and your child make will be more challenging than others, but just keep working on them. Remember, health is the greatest physical gift you can provide for your child, so every step forward through the program is a step in the right direction. If you get discouraged at any point, keep this in mind: Your child has one, and only one, body. The effort you invest in his physical health will be supremely rewarded.

What Is Your Body Saying?

Before you proceed, I want to mention one important thought: encourage your child to listen to her body! Your body would be considered astonishingly intelligent if it were viewed as a machine. If any food or supplement taken makes you or your child nauseated or sick in any way, it is very important to stop ingesting it immediately. Your body knows what is good for it. Most people, after adjusting to these nutritional recommendations, notice improvement in the way they feel after a few days or weeks. If this is not the case for you or your child, please consult a knowledgeable nutritional healthcare professional who understands insulin and fat biochemistry to help fine-tune your child's individual program.

Assessing Your Child's *Four Factors*

Although there is plenty of controversy and disagreement in medicine and nutritional science; most healthcare practitioners agree on four time-tested, clinically proven gauges that help determine a person's level of health:

- Insulin levels
- Weight
- Blood pressure
- Cholesterol levels

Like guideposts on a highway, these four factors direct you on the quest for wellness. Use them periodically to monitor your child's success on the Beginner Nutrition Plan.

Factor #1: Your Child's Insulin Level

We're all used to having our weight and blood pressure checked when we go to the doctor, but few people know their insulin level. I listed insulin level first in the Four Factors because it is so critical. Everyone needs insulin to live, but most of us have far too much of it in our bodies. I mentioned earlier in the book that the average adult's one gallon of blood typically contains only one teaspoon of sugar. If that same adult's blood-sugar level rose only to several tablespoons of sugar, they would quickly go into a hyperglycemic coma and die.

Your body produces insulin to keep your blood sugar at the appropriate level to keep you healthy. This is an important protective reflex response that literally keeps you from dying when you eat concentrated sugars. But too much of any good thing is typically associated with side effects, and that is clearly the case with insulin. Elevated levels of insulin are toxic for your body. If your child is overweight, you can be confident that any time he eats grains or sugars, he is increasing his insulin levels.

These increased insulin levels can eventually lead to all sorts of chronic diseases, such as heart disease, cancer, arthritis, and diabetes. Please understand that when I mention diabetes in this book I am normally referring to the most common type, type 2 diabetes. This type of diabetes is associated with increased weight and insulin resistance. Type 2 diabetes used to be called adult-onset diabetes because it typically occurred only in adults. However, troubling statistics indicate this type of diabetes is on the rise among children. Most children develop type 1 diabetes (previously called insulin-dependent diabetes), which results from lower-than-adequate insulin levels in the body, as the pancreas loses the ability to produce it.

Fasting blood-sugar and insulin test. To determine your child's blood-sugar levels, ask your doctor to perform a fasting blood-sugar test, also called an FBS, glucose test, or blood-sugar level test. A small amount of blood is withdrawn after a fasting period of six hours. It would also be helpful to have a blood-insulin level drawn at this time. Both of these tests are very inexpensive. I frequently find it more helpful than a blood-sugar level, as most of the time blood-sugar levels are normal in children, while they might have very elevated blood-insulin levels.

What these tests can tell you. A normal fasting blood sugar (FBS) should be around 87 mg/dL. Abnormal levels are cause for alarm. When the blood sugar rises above 110 mg/dL, it is called pre-diabetes. However, any fasting blood sugar over 100 is a strong indication that your sugar metabolism is not running properly.

Blood-sugar levels greater than 100 suggest insulin resistance and an inability to control blood-sugar levels. Left unchanged, this is a strong risk factor for developing diabetes in the future, as many as ten or more years down the road. With this extended early warning, there is plenty of time to make the appropriate nutritional and lifestyle changes necessary to avert the health disaster of diabetes.

A high fasting blood sugar is a strong indication that your child's insulin levels are too high. In addition, chronically high blood-sugar levels can accelerate the aging process of the body. When monitoring your child's Four Factors, look for FBS levels below 90.

When evaluating the fasting insulin levels, please understand that the reference ranges from the lab are based on "normals" of a population that has highly disturbed insulin levels, so you can safely ignore them. Here are my recommendations: A fasting insulin level should be 5 or below—the lower the better. A fasting insulin level above 10 suggests profound insulin disturbances; the higher the number, the worse. Levels above 20 are usually associated with people who are already diabetic.

Because grains have a profound effect on insulin levels, it is best to normalize your child's weight and exercise first before reintroducing grains back into their diet. Even then, grain consumption should be much lower than it was before starting the Total Health Program.

Factor #2: Your Child's Ideal Weight

Ideal weight is such a critical factor for optimal health that it motivated the writing of this book. About 27 percent of the world's population (or 1.7 billion people) are overweight, and the percentage just keeps going up.[1]

A very simple way to learn whether your child has a weight problem is to find out his waist circumference. Using an ordinary tape measure, measure the distance around the smallest area below the rib cage and above the belly button. This simple process measures total body fat more effectively than BMI (body mass index)—and it is also the best simple indicator of intra-abdominal fat mass.

BMI is useful for finding out what your child's ideal weight should be. The Centers for Disease Control has a good BMI calculator (http://www.cdc.gov/nccdphp/dnpa/bmi). Please note, however, that BMI is used differently for children than it is for adults. In children and teens, body mass index is used to assess the condition of being underweight, overweight, and at risk for being overweight. Children's body fatness changes as they grow and also differs between the genders. This is why BMI for children, also referred to as BMI-for-age, is gender- and age-specific. Typically, BMI decreases during the preschool years and then increases into adulthood.

Each of the CDC's gender-specific charts contains a series of curved lines indicating specific percentiles. Most healthcare professionals use the following percentile cutoff points to identify underweight and overweight children:

Underweight   BMI-for-age < 5th percentile

At risk of being overweight   BMI-for-age 85th percentile
                                       to < 95th percentile

Overweight   BMI-for-age ≥ 95th percentile

BMI example. The CDC gives the following example of BMI for a boy as he grows. While his BMI changes, he remains at the 95th percentile BMI-for-age.

AGE	BMI	PERCENTILE
2 years	19.3	95th
4 years	17.8	95th
9 years	21.0	95th
13 years	25.1	95th

This chart shows how the boy's BMI declines during his preschool years and increases as he gets older—meaning he is at a chronic state of being overweight.

(You can consult the gender-specific growth charts found at the CDC Web site for more information.)

I cannot overstate how important your child's ideal weight is for their overall health. Achieving that ideal weight is one of the primary goals of this book. Extra body weight can have far-reaching negative effects that follow your child into adulthood, both physically and emotionally. By helping your child achieve her ideal weight, you give her a powerful foothold on physical and psychological health that will serve her well in the future.

Factor #3: Your Child's Ideal Blood Pressure:

The American Academy of Pediatrics recommends that blood pressure be checked as part of the yearly checkup beginning at age three. In general, blood pressure normally increases as the child gets older. And blood pressure is also significantly affected by height, with the taller child having a higher blood pressure.

AGE	UPPER LIMIT OF SYSTOLIC BLOOD PRESSURE FOR BOYS	UPPER LIMIT OF DIASTOLIC BLOOD PRESSURE FOR BOYS
1	98–106	55–59
2	101–110	59–63
3	104–113	63–67
4	106–115	66–71
5	108–116	69–74
6	109–117	72–76
7	110–119	74–78
8	111–120	75–80
9	113–121	76–81
10	114–123	77–82
11	116–125	78–83
12	119–127	79–83
13	121–130	79–84
14	124–132	80–85
15	127–135	81–86
16	129–138	83–87
17	132–140	85–89

AGE	UPPER LIMIT OF SYSTOLIC BLOOD PRESSURE FOR GIRLS	UPPER LIMIT OF DIASTOLIC BLOOD PRESSURE FOR GIRLS
1	101–107	57–60
2	102–109	61–65
3	104–110	65–68
4	105–111	67–71
5	107–113	69–73
6	108–114	71–75
7	110–116	73–76
8	112–118	74–78
9	114–120	75–79
10	116–122	77–80
11	118–124	78–81
12	120–126	79–82
13	121–128	80–84
14	123–130	81–85
15	124–131	82–86
16	125–132	83–86
17	126–132	83–86

If your child's blood pressure is outside the ranges listed above, he has high blood pressure. If your child is on medication for high blood pressure, the good news is that this nutrition plan helps bring elevated blood pressures back into balance for the vast majority of people.

While elevated insulin levels are a potent contributor to elevated blood pressure, stress, tension, or anxiety can also contribute to this problem. After several months on the Total Health Program, your child should show an improvement in blood pressure. If not, please consult with a healthcare professional who is well-versed in using effective stress-relief methods.

Factor #4: Your Child's Ideal Cholesterol Level

Unfortunately, there is much confusion regarding cholesterol levels in our culture. Most people don't fully appreciate the importance of the relationship between the good and the bad or total cholesterol. The ratio, or relationship between the numbers, is actually a far more powerful predictor of heart disease than either value by itself.

To obtain the percentage of HDL, divide the HDL by the total cholesterol (HDL/Total Cholesterol). Ideally, this number should be above 24 percent. Levels below 10 percent are very dangerous and usually indicate an imminent cardiovascular problem. This number rarely gets above 50 percent, but to the best of my knowledge, the higher the number, the lower your risk of future cardiovascular disease.

Please note that some experts perform this calculation the other way around (Total Cholesterol/HDL). It provides the same information and is just as powerful, but one must use different numbers to evaluate. The cutoff point for a poor ratio would be any number greater than four; greater than ten indicates serious problems. This number rarely drops below two. I find it easier to use the HDL/Total Cholesterol, as it seems a more-logical view.

If your child rates high on the good-to-overall-cholesterol ratio, be encouraged: in my clinical experience the vast majority of people with a high cholesterol or triglyceride level rapidly respond to reducing their grains and sugars. This is especially true for triglycerides. In more than twenty years of practicing medicine, I have never seen an elevated triglyceride level fail to drop in response to someone who was compliant with a low-grain program.

Beginner Nutrition Plan

Again, one of the most important principles in the quest for health is to teach your child to listen to her body. If any food or supplement makes your child sick in any way, please have her stop ingesting it immediately. By teaching your child to actively "listen" to her body clues, you and your child will become experts at deciphering body language. I strongly believe that this is the primary feedback tool God gave each and every one of us. If you work on developing this skill, you can optimize your diet without having to consult expensive healthcare professionals.

Step 1: At Least One-Third of Your Child's Food Should Be Uncooked

There are valuable and sensitive micronutrients that are damaged when you heat foods. Cooking and processing food can destroy these highly sensitive and perishable micronutrients by altering their shape and chemical composition. Regular vegetable juicing can be a helpful tool for achieving this goal of one-third raw food in your diet.

Step 2: Eat More Vegetables

Let us first start out by describing how your child can and would definitely benefit from eating more vegetables. Vegetables promote health, unless your child is allergic to them or they cause gas or intestinal problems. Consult my "Recommended Vegetables" list below for the healthiest choices.

Recommended Vegetables:

asparagus	escarole
avocado (actually a fruit)	fennel
beet greens	green and red cabbage
bok choy	kale
broccoli	kohlrabi
brussels sprouts	lettuce: romaine, red leaf, green leaf
cauliflower	mustard greens
celery	onions
chicory	parsley
Chinese cabbage	peppers: red, green, yellow, and hot
chives	tomatoes
collard greens	turnips
dandelion greens	spinach
endive	zucchini

Avoid Eating Large Quantities of the Following if Insulin Levels Are Elevated:

beets	jicima
carrots	winter squashes
eggplant	potatoes

It would be best for your child to consume uncooked vegetables, but you may have to lightly steam them initially. Vegetables contain phytochemicals, which are powerful natural agents that promote health. They will also help to alkalinize your system, as most of us are far too acidic.

Your child normally requires a large amount of vegetables to stabilize his body's pH acid/alkaline balance and also to build strong bones and muscles. Although I will devote an entire chapter to vitamins and other supplements, your child will benefit more from increased vegetable consumption than from extra vitamins.

Each metabolic type has specific nutritional requirements, as we will learn in the next chapter, but nearly everyone benefits from the regular consumption of raw fresh vegetables. At the same time, remember that your child's body knows best and will tell you what is an optimal amount for her to eat. For example, because of differences in their genetic makeup, an Inuit child can't eat as many vegetables as can a Peruvian Indian child. If he did, he would feel bad and likely develop a ravenous appetite matched only by his sweet cravings.[2]

While we all need vegetables to stay healthy, the type and amount should be determined by our metabolic type. The basic metabolic-type test found in chapter 7 will give you a jump start in the process of identifying your metabolic type. Carbohydrate metabolic types need far more vegetables in their diet than protein metabolic types. Once you've established a dietary plan that has adequate vegetable servings for your child's metabolic type, let his young body report back to you how accurate his appetite/taste buds are at gauging what is right for him.

Step 3: Eat Organic Produce When Possible

Organic vegetables are best whenever practically possible, as not only are they free of harmful pesticides, but many studies show them to have up to three or four times as many nutrients as nonorganic vegetables. We will discuss this in greater detail in chapter 9. If you are unable to obtain them, you can rinse nonorganic vegetables in a sink full of water with four to eight ounces of distilled vinegar for thirty minutes.

Step 4: Keep Your Vegetables Fresh

Even the best organic vegetables will not provide you with many health benefits if they are spoiled. One of the easiest and least expensive things you can do in this area is make sure you remove as much air as possible out of the plastic bag in which you store the vegetables. You can do this by holding the bag with the vegetables against your chest with the open side up. Then roll your free arm across the bottom of the bag upward. This action forces the air out of the bag. Once you reach the top, secure the bag with a tie. Hopefully, you have a bag that looks like it was vacuum-packed. Room air is about 20 percent oxygen, and the oxygen will easily destroy the vegetables. When you remove the oxygen as described here, you can keep some of your vegetables fresh in the refrigerator for up to three weeks.

Step 5: Limit Your Child's Sugar Intake

If you're already familiar with the Total Health Program, you know that eliminating sugar ranks high on my list of "must" changes. Eating refined sugar weakens your child's immune system and promotes yeast overgrowth. All nondiet colas have eight teaspoons in each can. Most packaged cereals also have sugar as their major ingredient. I recommend that you avoid most natural sweeteners (including corn syrup, fructose, honey, sucrose, maltodextrin, dextrose, molasses, rice milk, almond milk, white grape juice, sweetened fruit juice, brown rice syrup, maple syrup, date sugar, cane sugar, corn sugar, beet sugar, succanat, and lactose).

A good rule of thumb for checking a food's sugar content is as follows: Look at the list of ingredients in the nutritional information box and see how many grams of carbohydrates are listed. Unless the carbohydrates are from aboveground vegetables, they most likely represent sugars. Since sugar directly affects insulin levels, you'll want to monitor your child's intake carefully.

OBESITY IMPAIRS IMMUNE RESPONSE OF MICE

Obesity apparently reduces laboratory mice's ability to turn on elements of their immune systems needed for controlling influenza infection, a new University of North Carolina at Chapel Hill School of Medicine study shows. The findings raise the possibility that obesity in humans has a similar effect, scientists say.

Compared to other mice of normal weight, which were otherwise identical, obese mice were ten times as likely to die when infected with the flu virus. Four percent of lean mice died during the experiments, compared with 40 percent of the extra-fat ones.

The study, presented in San Diego (April 2, 2005) at an American Society of Nutritional Sciences scientific gathering, which was part of a larger experimental biology meeting, was the first of its kind to examine the effects of obesity on the immune response to infection with influenza. Nutrition doctoral student Alexia Smith and Dr. Melinda A. Beck, associate

---

professor of pediatrics at the UNC School of Medicine, led the research and reported the findings.

"Numerous marked alterations seen in the mice's immune response suggest that the growing obese population is at increased risk for immune dysfunction during influenza infection, which may lead in humans, as it did in the mice, to increased mortality," Beck said.

". . . Another important finding was the reduced ability of natural killer cells in the obese animals," she said. "Natural killer cells are another central component of the early immune response. They limit viral replication by killing infected cells and have been shown to be important in the development of the T-cell response to influenza."

Natural killer cells in the obese animals had a 50 percent reduction in their killing capacity compared to lean animals, Beck said.[3]

Step 6: Avoid Hypoglycemia

Most of us eat large amounts of grains and sugars that generate a surplus of insulin in our blood. As a parent, be aware that when your child stops eating grains her body will take several days to lower its insulin levels. In the meantime her high insulin levels will cause symptoms such as dizziness, confusion, and headaches.

To avoid this temporary side effect, make sure your child eats every two hours for the first few days of the transition from her old eating pattern. It will be helpful to give her some food every ninety minutes to two hours for the first three days on the program. This will help prevent hypoglycemia and stabilize her blood sugar. You can have her eat a protein, such as an egg, a piece of chicken, turkey, fish, or some seeds, along with a nonstarchy vegetable.

Even after your child's system has adjusted, it will be wise to have her eat four to six meals a day. Eating more frequently, rather than consuming three large meals, helps to normalize cholesterol levels. It will also help her adrenal glands better regulate cortisol levels.

Because of my recommended avoidance of all dietary sugars, many people ask about using Equal® or NutraSweet® (aspartame) instead. Please understand that, in my opinion, artificial sweeteners are typically worse than sugar and need to be eliminated. I have written an entire book on this topic (*Sweet Deception*, Thomas Nelson, 2006).

More adverse reactions from NutraSweet are reported to the FDA than all other foods and additives combined.[4] If your child is healthy, allow them to use a few teaspoons of succanat here and there. I also recommend avoiding artificial chemicals like MSG.

Menus lead to success. You may have heard the adage "Those who fail to plan, plan to fail." Making a new start on healthy eating is a challenge for most people, and if you don't plan your meals, you may be shooting yourself in the foot. To guarantee success on the Total Health Program, it will be helpful to you to sit down once a week and plan your child's meals for the week ahead.

Many with full-time jobs often find that preparing the family's meals ahead of time helps. For example, you could make your child's lunch for the next day before you go to bed. Knowing what you will eat for dinner before you leave the house in the morning is a great strategy to stay ahead of the game. This way you can go to the store or take the appropriate items out of the freezer. Those who don't do this more easily slip back into their old, less-healthy eating habits. Sit down with your child and together find ten recipes that you like. You may have to experiment a little before finding the right recipes—ones that you and your family enjoy—but that is just part of the process. You can even make it into a game of sorts, trying this and that recipe until you arrive at a top ten list.

After nutritional content, variety is the most important aspect of meal planning. If you rotate only two or three different meals, your child (and/or family) will burn out and stop the program. Variety is the key.

Step 7: Emotional Food Cravings Can Masquerade as Physical Food Cravings—Learn the Difference

With the glut of fad diet advice on the market today, most people are familiar with the term "emotional eating." In short, emotional eating is stuffing your body full of feel-good foods to compensate for some (emotional) area of life that doesn't feel good. If your child still craves sweets or grains after the weaning process, you will need to determine if their cravings are emotionally based.

Many people don't understand that emotional well-being is essential to physical health. In fact, not addressing emotional issues—small or serious traumas from the past—is the primary reason why most people who lose weight gain it all back. A child who is bogged down with negative thoughts and feelings about himself will typically not succeed at weight loss. The energy consumed by negativity saps the effort required to make nutritional changes. You can compare it to washing your car in a dust storm. Resetting the brain to "positive" mode is imperative if your child hopes to achieve optimal physical health. Chapter 10 includes many practical strategies you can implement to help you overcome these barriers to success.

DISCOVER YOUR CHILD'S METABOLIC TYPE

7

The goal of this book is to help you optimize your child's health and normalize his or her weight. Along with that two-pronged goal is a third component that I consider a nonnegotiable for overall health: abundant energy.

One of the most important actions you can take to optimize your child's health is to begin the process of identifying your child's metabolic type so you can feed them foods in the proper ratios. What is healthy and nutritionally ideal for other kids may not be as healthy for your child, and vice versa. Metabolic typing will teach you the best foods for your child's specific genetic heritage, foods that will fight and prevent disease and improve the way your child feels physically and emotionally. To acquire a better understanding of how and why metabolic typing works, let's return to our car analogy.

The Right Fit, the Right Fuel

Just as food is fuel for our bodies, gas is food for our cars. Suppose you buy a new car and pull into a high-end gas station that offers the best-quality gasoline from one of the world's leading refineries. The station owner assures you his gas is free of anything that could possibly harm your car's engine.

Without knowing any other details, you might reasonably assume the car will thrive on that high-quality gas. But what if you neglected to find out one crucial detail about your car—namely, that it's a diesel-powered vehicle? A few minutes down the road your car would stop running, and you would have a very expensive repair job ahead of you.

The fact that the car stopped running does not imply that the gas wasn't good or that your car was defective. It was simply the wrong type of fuel for your car. Like a car, your child's body was designed for a certain type of fuel—that is, a certain correct blend of the right food types. The further he deviates from this ideal, the more health problems your child is likely to endure.

I can't tell you how many sick people come through the door of my clinic who eat nothing but "health foods." The problem is, they are eating health foods that are good for other people, but not for them. Those who are designed to be eating high-protein foods may have decided to be vegetarians. Or perhaps they are carb types but they have determined a diet of high protein is best—and then suffer for it.

Eating foods that are right for your child's metabolic type should produce marked improvement in their energy, mental capacity, and emotional well-being. They should also feel well-satisfied for several hours.

If your child already feels good, proper eating should help to maintain that energy level. But if he feels worse an hour or so after eating, or if he:

- still feels hungry even though he is physically full,

- develops a sweet craving,

- experiences a drop in energy level, or

- feels hyper, nervous, angry, irritable, or depressed,

then there is a good chance it might be due to an improper ratio of proteins, fats, and carbohydrates at his last meal. Your child might be eating the right foods for his metabolic type, but having too much of one type of food in place of another can easily produce the symptoms listed above.

Discover Your Child's Unique Metabolic Type

The metabolic typing questionnaire found in this chapter will help you determine which of three general metabolic types your child falls under:

- Protein

- Carb

- Mixed

We will cover the basics of metabolic typing here in *Generation XL*, but if you desire an in-depth look at biochemistry and why it is crucial to optimizing your child's health and weight, I suggest reading *The Metabolic Typing Diet* by William Wolcott, one of the pioneers of metabolic typing. Wolcott's book also contains another metabolic typing test you can use.

Making Sense of the Different Metabolic Types

As the name implies, protein types do better on diets low in carbohydrates but high in protein and fats. A typical ratio might be 40 percent protein and 30 percent each of fats and carbohydrates, but the amounts could easily shift to 50 percent fats and as little as 10 percent carbohydrates, depending on individual genetic requirements.

Carb types function best when a majority of their diet comes from carbohydrates—typically as much as 60 percent. However, there are many different types of carbohydrates. Vegetables and grains are radically different foods—and have different effects on the body—and yet they are both referred to as carbs.

Not understanding the distinction between grains and vegetables is a prescription for health troubles. Over two-thirds of Americans are overweight or obese, and nearly every one of these individuals needs to lower their insulin levels. Eliminating or greatly reducing grain consumption is the easiest way to do that. Most people with high blood pressure, high cholesterol, and diabetes also struggle with elevated insulin levels—and all three health problems respond well to grain restriction. It is safe to say that over 85 percent of the U.S. population would benefit from a low-grain or grain-free diet, not a low-carb diet, such as the South Beach or Atkins Diet.

So if your child is a carb metabolic type, about 60 percent of her food should be carbs, 25 percent protein, and 15 percent fat. Sometimes carb types need as little as 10 percent fat and as high as 80 percent carbs. If the same child followed one of the popular "low-carb" diets, she might improve for a while, but eventually her system would break down because it required far more carbohydrates.

Let me stress that once a person attains an ideal weight (and does not have other insulin-related disorders), he can usually consume some whole grains and remain perfectly healthy. Carb types can actually do quite well with whole grains as long as their insulin levels are normal.

Mixed metabolic types require foods from both the carb and protein type dietary lists, and some customizing will likely be involved. The good news is that they can eat just about any healthy food. The bad news is that they need to pay much more attention to what their bodies are telling them as a guide to the right food choices. As a parent, you will have to rely heavily on feedback gathered from answering the questions after every meal. Please don't stress out about the percentages; they are only rough guidelines. Just do the best you can.

Keep in mind that your child's activity and stress levels will also affect the quantity of food—as well as the ratio of proteins, fats, and carbohydrates—she needs to feel her best. Finally, take into account the very real issue of circadian rhythm. Every human being's biochemistry moves through various phases throughout the day. These rhythms involve hormonal output, acid/alkaline shifts, waking/sleeping times, and many other time-based variables. While some people do well on the same ratios of protein, fat, and carbs at each meal, others need different ratios at different meals to feel their best.

Getting Started

As you move into the Beginner phase of the Total Health Program, you'll find that it is really quite simple and straightforward. Here's a generalized overview of how to begin:

Start by having your child eat the proportions of proteins, fats, and carbs according to their taste and appetite. Next, analyze his reactions to each meal and learn how well you did in selecting the right ratios for him. Older children can learn to do this for themselves.

Finally, if your child did not react optimally to his meal, change the ratios the next time he eats that meal and analyze his reactions. This is the best way to fine-tune each meal to the ratio of proteins, fats, and carbs that is just right for your child.

Let me provide a personal example of how these ratios can make a difference. I used to have a salad with turkey in it for lunch. However, not long after, I would feel famished and fight strong food cravings all afternoon. As you know, the largest part of turkey is white meat. Well, white meat is very low in fat, and that is what I was eating most of the time. Additionally, I was not using a high-fat salad dressing. So my fat content for the meal was probably south of 10 percent. Once I learned about metabolic typing, it was quite obvious that I needed more fat (about 40 percent) for lunch. So I still had a salad, but I used ground beef or dark chicken or turkey meat with plenty of olive oil, and my food cravings disappeared.

Remember that your child should feel terrific one hour after they eat. Food cravings or decreased energy levels are giant clues that he is not eating correctly for his metabolic type. Before taking the metabolic typing test, realize that *learning your child's metabolic type is essential if you want to optimize his health and weight for the long haul.* Why? Just as your child is unique in all other respects, his body has a unique biochemistry requiring certain proportions and types of healthy carbohydrates, fats, and proteins.

Metabolic typing is not a quick fix; it requires a measure of discipline and stick-to-itiveness. At the same time, it is a proven dietary principle that has been used for decades with astonishing results. I have employed it with thousands of patients in my Optimal Wellness Center, helping patients overcome severe chronic disease, obesity, and other serious disorders.

Learning your child's metabolic type will help clear up the dietary "mysteries" you may have struggled with, including these:

- Why can some people lose weight—at least in the short term—on popular low-carb, low-fat, or other popular diets, while many others fail miserably on the very same diet from the get-go?

- Why is it that one type of food can be so good for one person and so bad for another, making her tired, cranky, or feeling otherwise unwell?

Learning your child's correct metabolic type and fine-tuning his diet will clear up these "mysteries" and many more. Best of all, it will optimize his ability to fight and prevent disease and achieve his ideal weight by measures that will astound you.

Answer the questions included in the test (for or with your child), choosing the number on the scale beneath each question that most accurately reflects your child's response. There are no right or wrong answers, and if you aren't sure about any given question, just go with your hunches.

This basic-level test is a useful first step toward identifying the types and proportions of macronutrients that are ideal for your child. His metabolic type will be automatically determined at the conclusion of the test. Please understand that the ONLY purpose of the basic test is to give you a starting point. It is not designed as a definitive tool to permanently label your child with a specific metabolic type. This is not possible because your child's metabolic type can be relatively dynamic.

Extreme carb or protein types rarely change their metabolic type, but most everyone else seems to shift back and forth. It is typically only a one-category shift. So a protein might become a mixed or a mixed might shift to a carb. It is very uncommon for a protein to shift to a carb type or vice versa. Variables like the time of year, activity levels, and stress can cause this shift.

It is probably more useful to view metabolic typing as a process or a journey in which you are constantly challenging your body with different ratios of foods and listening to your body to find out which combinations and ratios make you and your child feel best. I strongly believe that the table following the test, which will help you listen to your body, is far more valuable than the test below.

Basic Metabolic Type Test

The following test will help jump-start the process of determining your child's metabolic type. Please understand that it is only a starting point. You will need to answer the questions in the table to ultimately confirm the result.

It is important to reiterate that this test is a very condensed version of the sophisticated and expansive computerized Intermediate version that was designed by William Wolcott over a period of thirty years. Metabolic type exists on a spectrum; while the computerized version is more accurate, this abbreviated version still provides a reasonable point from which to launch your deeper understanding of your child's type and fine-tuning her diet.

For the following general test, simply choose the number that best represents your answer on the scale provided for each question.

Question 1:
Does a high-carbohydrate meal or snack, one that is loaded with plenty of vegetables, bread, toast, cereals, rice, fruits, grains, or potatoes as the main food source, satisfy your child's appetite or stimulate it further?

○ 1 ○ 2 ○ 3 ○ 4 ○ 5 ○ 6 ○ 7 ○ 8 ○ 9 ○ 10

Satisfies   *Stimulates*

Question 2:

When your child eats a lot of red meat, does it cause her to lose or gain body fat? Does she look slimmer in the mirror, or is it easier for her clothes to fit?

○ 1 ○ 2 ○ 3 ○ 4 ○ 5 ○ 6 ○ 7 ○ 8 ○ 9 ○ 10
Gain Weight   *Lose Weight*

Question 3:

Does your child constantly think about food and frequently look forward with eager anticipation to his next meal or what he wants to eat?

○ 1 ○ 2 ○ 3 ○ 4 ○ 5 ○ 6 ○ 7 ○ 8 ○ 9 ○ 10
No   *Yes*

Question 4:

What is your child's appetite like at breakfast, lunch, and dinner?

Breakfast

○ 1 ○ 2 ○ 3 ○ 4 ○ 5 ○ 6 ○ 7 ○ 8 ○ 9 ○ 10
Weaker   *Stronger*

Lunch

○ 1 ○ 2 ○ 3 ○ 4 ○ 5 ○ 6 ○ 7 ○ 8 ○ 9 ○ 10
Weaker   *Stronger*

Dinner

○ 1 ○ 2 ○ 3 ○ 4 ○ 5 ○ 6 ○ 7 ○ 8 ○ 9 ○ 10
Weaker   *Stronger*

Question 5:

Does eating something higher in fat and/or protein such as dark meats, avocados, cream, butter, or coconuts within an hour or two of bedtime help your child to sleep better?

○ 1 ○ 2 ○ 3 ○ 4 ○ 5 ○ 6 ○ 7 ○ 8 ○ 9 ○ 10
Yes   *No*

Question 6:

If your child ate a large salad with some low-fat meat like chicken breast for lunch (versus a higher-fat meat like a hamburger patty), how would it affect his energy level throughout the rest of the afternoon?

○ 1 ○ 2 ○ 3 ○ 4 ○ 5 ○ 6 ○ 7 ○ 8 ○ 9 ○ 10

Ample energy and hunger satisfied   *Become tired and hungry*

Question 7:

How often does your child typically feel the need to eat on an average day? The extremes here would be feeling good with one meal scored as a 1, while needing five or six meals a day would place them at a 10. Feeling good on three meals a day would be a 5.

○ 1 ○ 2 ○ 3 ○ 4 ○ 5 ○ 6 ○ 7 ○ 8 ○ 9 ○ 10

Feels good on 1–2 meals,   *Feels good on 5–6 meals,*
including snacks   *including snacks*

Question 8:

How much does your child enjoy sour foods like pickles, sauerkraut, or vinegar?

○ 1 ○ 2 ○ 3 ○ 4 ○ 5 ○ 6 ○ 7 ○ 8 ○ 9 ○ 10

Loves them   *Can't stand them*

Question 9:

At Thanksgiving or a meal where your child eats turkey, and assuming all the turkey is moist, if she prefers white meat, give her a 1; if she prefers the dark meat, give her a 10; and if it doesn't matter, give her a 5.

○ 1 ○ 2 ○ 3 ○ 4 ○ 5 ○ 6 ○ 7 ○ 8 ○ 9 ○ 10

Prefers white meat   *Prefers dark meat*

Now add up the eleven numbers you marked to get your child's total score and basic metabolic type:

- A score over 60 indicates a Protein Type. The higher the score above 60, the more likely your child is truly a Protein Type.

- A score under 60 indicates a Carb Type. The lower the score under 60, the more likely your child is truly a Carb Type.

- A score between 40 and 70 indicates a potential Mixed Type. If your child scored in this range, you can begin fine-tuning her diet as explained below, but it is recommended that you take the more-sophisticated test in William Wolcott's book, *The Metabolic Typing Diet*, to provide yourself a more reliable starting point.

First, because the test you just took provides a basic estimate of your child's metabolic type, you will want to do the following:

1. Use your child's MT test results as a starting point for honing in much closer to his body's particular biochemical requirements for the right **proportions** of carbohydrates, proteins, and fats.

2. Learn the healthiest **forms** of the carbohydrates, proteins, and fats, including (and this is critical) *the healthiest forms for your child's particular metabolic type*, as the foods that may be beneficial for his type are not necessarily healthy for other types. See the second chart on page 86, "Some Recommended Foods for Each Metabolic Type."

The chart on page 86, "General Macronutrient Proportions for Each Metabolic Type," provides a standard macronutrient proportion guide to start from for each of the metabolic types. Each of the percentages represents the approximate amount of proteins, fats, and carbohydrates that each type should consume on a daily basis, *but* it is essential that you learn the principles of *listening* to your child's body and fine-tuning her diet to begin understanding how to use this chart.

In short, listening to your child's body requires paying attention to a variety of signals up to two hours after your child eats a meal in order to "hear" what her body is telling you about what she just ate. For instance, does your child feel her energy has been restored? Or instead, does she feel tired and lack energy?

These answers are signs that he is either eating the right proportions and forms of macronutrients for his body's biochemistry (leading to dramatically improved health and optimized weight), or he is eating proportions or forms of macronutrients that are not right for his metabolic type (leading to health and weight issues). Fine-tuning his diet, in short, means learning how to adjust your child's next meal, and his diet in general, based on "listening" to your child's body.

GENERAL MACRONUTRIENT PROPORTIONS FOR EACH METABOLIC TYPE	
Carb Type:	25% Protein / 15% Fat / 60% Carbohydrates
Mixed Type:	30% Protein / 20% Fat / 50% Carbohydrates
Protein Type:	40% Protein / 30% Fat / 30% Carbohydrates

SOME RECOMMENDED FOODS FOR EACH METABOLIC TYPE	
This is just a very short sampling of the foods that tend to be most beneficial for each type. Mixed types will benefit from many foods ideal for both carb and protein types, but in proportions according to their needs. *Dr. Mercola's Total Health Cookbook & Program* provides more-comprehensive lists that are essential references for all types.	
CARB OR MIXED TYPE	**PROTEIN OR MIXED TYPE**
• chicken breast	• beef (grass-fed)
• turkey breast	• turkey, dark meat
• Cornish game hen	• bison meat
• broccoli	• asparagus
• peppers	• spinach
• citrus fruits	• avocados
• tomatoes	• cauliflower

How to Customize Your Child's Diet

Analyze your child's responses to the different foods in her diet, making adjustments where necessary. This is an imperfect science, but the body is the best barometer of what is good for it. As you tweak your child's nutritional program, you will eventually find a custom fit that is ideal for her biochemistry.

Suppose an hour after lunch your son felt sleepy, hungry, and wanted some caffeine or something sweet. These are clear indications that the ratios at lunch were far off-kilter for his metabolism. Have him eat the same foods for lunch the next day but dramatically change the ratios. As a result of this change, your son will feel noticeably better—or worse. You'll know you are either on the right track or needing to go in the opposite direction with his ratios. In other words, if you dramatically increase his protein and lower his carbs, and his symptoms worsen, that means you need to lower his protein and increase his carbs.

The body knows best—far more than any diet expert ever will. It will always tell you exactly how well you did in providing what it needs, once you learn to interpret its "body language."

HOW TO HELP YOUR CHILD WANT GOOD FOOD

Children can be tough to feed—especially in our convenience-obsessed world. The tendency is to feed them the easy stuff—the food they will more readily like and that's more easily prepared. Most parents find it much easier first thing in the morning to open a box of sugared cereal and pour some milk on it than to take the time to soft-boil an egg.

However, remember that sugared cereal shaped like some sort of cartoon character contains so much sugar and so many colorings, preservatives, and chemicals, it is amazing kids even survive the morning. Forget about their sitting in school and trying to concentrate. It would be safer and more nutritious to feed them the box.

Kids need as much or more good food than adults do, and not less. While they may not like it as much as the sugary, fried, greasy, and colorful alternatives, eventually they will not only *eat* good food, but they will *ask* for it. By feeding them more natural foods, you will see them become more accustomed to the taste, and their addictions to salt and sugar will slowly diminish.

While parents often become concerned that their kids don't want nutritious foods and won't eat them, the reality is that kids will typically not allow themselves to starve. There are a few "tricks" I use to begin helping children understand how processed foods hurt them and why they should start eating fresh, healthy, unprocessed foods.

When I explain food colorings to children, I let them know that the colors are made up of much the same stuff as crayons and markers! When they understand that drinking an orange soda or eating a blue lollipop is like drinking an orange crayon or eating a blue pen, they are much less likely to reach for them.

I also like to read them the labels on their foods and then show them how some garage products or home and office supplies are made up of the same types of additives and preservatives. This is a great way to show them that eating ice cream, cookies, and fast food is a lot like drinking turpentine or drain cleaner, or eating pencil shavings!

Commercial fruit juice is a common kid filler used by parental units everywhere. The problem is that most fruit juices are pasteurized and filled with a lot more sugar than those you would fresh-squeeze at home. I would strongly discourage using any commercial fruit juices. Fruit juices are not the best fluid for your child, as they have loads of sugar. It would be far better to eat the whole fruit. However, if you are going to use fruit juices, it would be best to prepare them at home so your children are receiving the highest quality possible.

Snacks can be purchased from the health-food store. While these "treats" are still refined, they are not filled with many of the artificial ingredients that are present in most grocery stores.

If children become accustomed to good food, they will begin making better choices that will not only affect them for a lifetime but will actually *increase* their lifetimes. Let your kids know that good food is what they really want to eat—and tell them the truth about what "good" food really is. They feed their fish "fish food" and their dogs "dog food," so why not feed their own bodies "people food"?

LIQUID ASSETS: THE GOOD, BAD, AND UGLY OF BEVERAGES

8

Did you know that water makes up more than 70 percent of your body's tissues? Water plays a role in nearly every bodily function, from cushioning joints and regulating temperature to bringing oxygen to your cells and removing waste from your body. Someone once said, "You are what you eat," and it's equally true that you are what you drink. For that reason, making certain your child drinks enough clean water should be at the top of the list as you prioritize his or her new way of eating and living.

All the food categories mentioned in this book are important, but while your body can literally go for weeks without food, it can exist only a few days without water. Without water, your body sends a *system malfunction* red-alert message and eventually shuts down.

If you took all the water out of your body, you would basically be powder. Even at the cellular level, the body reflects the quality of fluids it takes in. Sources of poor drinking water such as nearly all municipal tap water, coffee, or soda dilute the quality of water in your body with chemicals, additives, toxins, and heavy metals. Your body requires clean water to continuously flush out the toxins and acids you consume and produce every day. A good rule of thumb about drinking water is this: never drink anything you wouldn't take a bath in!

Making the transition from drinking sodas to drinking nothing but water may take some time. Juice, whether fresh-squeezed or commercial, can serve as a happy medium. One of the best ways to ease the pain of this transition is to dilute half a pitcher of fruit juice with water. Gradually increase the water dilution over a period of a few weeks. As your child gets used to the increasingly diluted fruit juice, his taste buds will wean themselves to a state of accepting the watery flavor. The next step, of course, is to introduce them to pure, clean water.

To keep your child's internal hydration system running at peak efficiency—a level of fluids the body cells thrive in—have him drink plenty of water. But how much is *plenty*, you may be wondering. While it is unlikely that your child would ever drink too much water, it is very likely they are not drinking enough. And remember that the water they consume should contain two H's, an O, and as little else as possible!

Do You Really Need Eight Glasses of Water a Day?

Most of us have grown up hearing the traditional admonition to drink eight 8-ounce glasses of water a day. I used to advise that people follow an even-stricter rule of thumb—for every fifty pounds of body weight you carry, drink one quart of spring water or filtered water per day. This would increase daily water intake to twelve to sixteen glasses for most of us.

After a while, however, I refined my recommendations to a simple formula that uses the color of your urine as a guide to water intake. As long as you are not taking vitamin B_2 (riboflavin), which turns your urine bright yellow, your urine should be a very light-colored yellow. If it is a deep or dark yellow color, or worse, yellowish orange, you are simply not drinking enough water.

I firmly believe this is a superior way to monitor your water intake. It is in direct alignment with listening to your body's recommendations, and I believe it is a far more accurate approach than blindly drinking a rigid amount of water per day. It is important to trust that God gave you enough tools to figure this out for yourself. There are far too many variables in hydration to be tied to some rigid formula.

The same goes for your child. Monitor his morning urine (ask him not to flush after his first trip to the bathroom each day) to make sure he is getting an adequate supply of water in his system. School-age children can easily learn to do this for themselves, and you might even make it into a daily challenge of sorts.

An Institute of Medicine panel actually reached the same conclusion regarding water intake. The panel concluded that on a daily basis people get enough water from normal drinking behavior, such as drinking beverages at meals and in other social situations, and by letting their thirst guide them. The conventional wisdom of eight glasses of water a day appears to have been upstaged by this more natural—and, let's face it, more manageable—method of gauging water intake.

I do believe, though, for most of us the cumulative amount of clean water that we need is close to the proverbial eight glasses per day. But fine-tune that amount by listening to your body so it is perfect for you.

Listening to your body does not negate the need for a steady water supply to your body. Please carefully review the following list of water's vital functions in your body:

- Is essential for digestion, nutrient absorption, and elimination

- Aids circulation

- Helps control the body's temperature

- Lubricates and cushions joints

- Keeps the skin healthy

- Helps remove toxins from the body

Every day the human body loses water through urine and sweat, and this fluid needs to be replenished. Being the efficient machine that it is, however, the body has a built-in mechanism that tells you when you need to replenish your supply—it's called thirst!

Follow Your Thirst

Perhaps it sounds simplistic to say, "Let your thirst be your guide," but that is essentially all you need to do. When the body begins to lose 1–2 percent of its total water, your thirst mechanism lets you know it's time to drink some water. Now let's translate this to your child. If your child is healthy in all respects other than her weight, drinking whenever she feels thirsty should be an adequate guide of how much water she needs. Again, you can confirm whether she is drinking enough water by the color of her urine.

When the mercury soars on the thermometer, your body naturally perspires—losing a lot of water in the process. So if it's hot outside or your child is exercising or doing some other vigorous activity, he will require more water than normal. Be sure he stays well hydrated in these cases.

Fortunately, our thirst mechanism is at its peak in our youth, as this aspect of the body works less efficiently with age. (This is why I always recommend that older adults consume a steady supply of water—children have it a lot easier in this regard!)

Water, Water Everywhere—But Is It Good to Drink?

For too long we've been kicking around the question of how much water to drink, but perhaps the more-appropriate question is: what type of water should we be drinking? The answer is clean spring water and filtered water. Neither Dr. Lerner nor I recommend drinking most municipal tap waters or distilled water. And, contrary to what you may have thought, you should avoid fluoridated water as well.

I can hear you asking: But what about the dental health benefits of drinking fluoridated water? Doesn't my child need this? Fluoride is a substance that poisons your enzymes. You might already know that enzymes are important proteins in your body that facilitate or catalyze chemical reactions essential to your health. Even very low concentrations of fluoride can damage your enzymes and their functions. Further, fluoride from all sources (water, air, and food) accumulates in the body, which can only eliminate 50 percent of its total fluoride intake, causing harm to your immune system, musculoskeletal system, genes, and thyroid.

It is very important to ensure the safety of your tap-water supply by having it tested for contaminants by a reputable water-testing company. Doing so will help you determine what type of filter you need to rid your water of heavy metals, bacteria, and other harmful contaminants.

Because bottled water places such a significant strain on our environment, I am a major advocate of filtering your own water. Besides, some brands of bottled water are no cleaner than tap water. On a side note, remember to avoid storing your water in typical Nalgene bottles, as they can leach an unsafe chemical called BPA into your water. The high-density polyethelene (HDPE) Nalgene bottles appear to be a safer alternative and can be readily found at www.campmor.com.

Following are a handful of guidelines for your child's daily water intake:

Lesson 1: Have your child drink enough water so that her urine is a light yellow color on a consistent basis. We just covered this point extensively, so suffice it to say that drinking enough water is one of the simplest and most important health steps your child can take. If your child normally doesn't drink enough water, you'll have to build up her water intake gradually to prevent her running to the bathroom every few minutes. Her bladder will adjust to this higher water volume after a short period of time.

By drinking an adequate supply of water, your child can easily avoid dehydration, which can have profound negative effects on their health. Dehydration can cause the following symptoms:

- Fatigue

- Dry skin

- Headaches

- Constipation

Lesson 2: Make sure your child drinks water at the right pace. It's far better to sip water all day than to guzzle a quart all at once. Depending on your child's size, his body can process only a bit more than a glass of water per hour. If he drinks much more than this at one sitting, the extra water will not be used but merely flushed down the toilet bowl. A water bottle kept handy throughout the day is the best option. Most schoolteachers are now allowing students to keep water bottles at their desks, but if your child's teacher prohibits drinking of any kind during class, encourage your school-age child to sip from a water bottle (carried in his backpack) between classes or on bathroom breaks. You'll have to make reasonable adjustments for younger children.

Lesson 3: Drink healthy water. Don't be fooled! Not all water is healthy. In fact, most drinking water is only water that has been treated to avoid contamination. American municipal water supplies typically add chlorine and fluoride, although Europeans have long known that fluoride is toxic and removed it from their water supplies years ago. A good filter will help you avoid chlorine and fluoride.

Here's another unpleasant surprise: about 5 percent of our water supplies contain unhealthy arsenic levels, and arsenic, being a poison, can cause serious health problems.

Additionally, thousands of tons of drugs are flushed down the toilet each year. Since most filtration plants aren't designed to remove them, it's reasonable to conclude these drug residues may wind up in your water supply.

I recommend that you avoid distilled water. Evidence exists that this form of water has seriously adversely altered its molecular structure. Additionally, it has the wrong ionization, pH, polarization, and oxidation potentials. Distilled water also tends to drain your body of minerals. Although this is a controversial subject in natural-health circles, the evidence against using distilled water appears to outweigh arguments for it.

You have several options for obtaining healthy water in your home. Find and use the one that works best for your family:

Buy Bottled Spring water

Although bottled spring water is acceptable, it is expensive and disposing of all those plastic bottles also puts a strain on the environment. Think of how often you (may) drink bottled water and then multiply that amount by millions of other users. If you select the bottled-water option, it would be best to use the five-gallon bottles at home that are recycled.

Filter Your Water

I recommend two main types of filters:

- **Carbon filters:** These work well to remove impurities but may not remove fluoride. The PUR Faucet Mount Water Filter and the GE Smart Water Filter both get high marks from me. The GE model was top-rated in the *Consumer Reports* December 2002 issue.

- **Reverse-osmosis filters:** This type of water-purifying system removes most impurities. Reverse-osmosis filtration systems filter water by squeezing water through a semipermeable membrane, the same technology used to make bottled water, and they are capable of desalinating sea water, making it into drinking water.

Store Your Water Safely

The one-gallon cloudy plastic (PVC) containers from the grocery store transfer far too many chemicals into your water. The five-gallon containers and the clear bottles (polyethylene) are a much better plastic and will not give the water an unpalatable plastic taste.

Find an Economical Solution

PUR and Brita both offer high-quality water filtration. The PUR Faucet Mount Water Filter is a solid and economical choice, while Brita water-filtration pitchers are also a good choice. (Brita filters cost approximately twenty-four cents per gallon, while bottled water costs one to two dollars per gallon!)

Lesson 4: Use lemon or lime juice to add a bit of flavor and normalize your child's pH level. Adding lemon or lime juice to your child's water will not only help flavor it; doing so also normalizes his body's pH (alkaline/acidic balance). However, be careful not to use lemon juice continuously, or your child may develop an allergy to it.

Lesson 5: Assess your home water-delivery system. If you have a water softener, divert the softened water away from the kitchen tap to a reverse-osmosis system. If you have municipal water, attach filters to your bathroom shower-heads to remove the chlorine. Believe it or not, this exposure could actually be greater than exposure from drinking tap water. Those who draw their water supply from a well don't need to take this precaution. You can order a PUR Faucet Mount Water Filter online at http://www.purwater.com/products/ utlimate_vert.shtml. Brita filtration pitchers are available in most discount retailers such as Wal-Mart, Target, and Kmart. You can obtain reverse-osmosis systems locally from Home Depot or through Coast Filtration (800-542-6723).

Lesson 6: Monitor all other fluids.

Coffee and Tea

In the Beginner nutrition level, your child can have unlimited tea; some older children may even drink coffee. If they struggle with insomnia or anxiety, however, you should have them avoid all caffeine.

A Word About Caffeine

Caffeine is a common stimulant found in everything from chocolate and colas to herbs and medication. Many people use it to raise their normal energy levels in the morning—it's been called the "last legal drug." This process is repeated to keep them awake throughout the day so that by the next morning it has to be started all over again. What a vicious cycle!

Your body is always seeking homeostasis, or a natural balance of function and physiology. If you drink or swallow something that elevates your body's power level, you cause a disturbance in this balance, and the body tries to save itself by bringing power levels back down. Over time, the body keeps adjusting its natural power state downward to compensate for this overstimulation.

That is why it eventually takes more and more caffeine to give you any effect. Sooner or later you have to drink a soda or cup of coffee just to get back to "tired."

As with all stimulants, every time you drink caffeine, you affect your heart function, alter your vascular flow, and overstimulate digestive and glandular activity. Anytime you manipulate your body in any way, you end up throwing off your normal energy balance, which can eventually cause organ system failure and glandular meltdown. The regular use of caffeine or any material that speeds up your body function will ultimately slow it down.

Juices

Fruit juices are also allowed in the Beginner level, but as we mentioned earlier, seek to limit (and dilute) them as much as possible, as they contain large amounts of sugar.

Avoid All Soft Drinks!

From my perspective, there is no justifiable reason for anyone to drink soft drinks ever—period. For every can of soda that a child drinks per day, his or her risk of obesity increases by 60 percent.[1]

Drink Only Raw, Unpasteurized Cow's Milk

Commercial milk goes through a processing and refining system known as "pasteurization." During pasteurization, the milk is heated to kill off germs. The high heat changes the actual three-dimensional shape of the proteins in the milk. Once changed, these new, altered proteins, especially casein, can cause allergic reactions and contribute to many autoimmune diseases.

Pasteurizing milk destroys enzymes, diminishes vitamins, denatures fragile milk proteins, destroys vitamin B_{12} and vitamin B_6, kills beneficial bacteria, and promotes pathogens. You may notice that raw milk left out will sour naturally, but pasteurized milk will rot. This is because the beneficial bacteria in the raw milk helps to keep putrefactive bacteria under control. Pasteurized milk, however, does not have any of the beneficial bacteria left to keep it from rotting.

It is far more important to use raw milk than organic milk, as most organic milk is not raw and the major problems from milk result from its pasteurization, not the addition of synthetic chemicals and hormones. However, it still is important to have hormone- and antibiotic-free milk; you just need to understand that the pasteurization is a more central issue.

Except for a brief gap in 1990, raw milk has always been for sale commercially in California, usually in health-food stores, although previously it was even sold in regular grocery stores. Millions of people consumed commercial raw milk during that period, and although the health department kept an eagle eye open for any possible evidence of harm, not a single incidence was reported. During the same period, there were many instances of contamination in pasteurized milk, some of which resulted in death.

Unless you live in California, it will be very difficult to obtain raw milk. The simplest way would be to find a farmer who is willing to sell it to you. Many farmers are concerned about legal issues. A easy way to work around this problem is what is called a "cow share" program, in which you purchase a portion of the farmer's cow for ten dollars. This allows the farmer to legally milk your cow for you. In my practice we have a group of Amish farmers who travel several hundred miles every week to and from Michigan to provide the patients in our practice access to this amazing health food.

Ideally, the milk should be from cows that are not factory-farmed but humanely raised and fed primarily grass. Fortunately, most of the dairy farmers who are clued into the benefits of raw milk also understand the importance of excluding grains, antibiotics, and pesticides from their dairy cows' diet. So if you find cows that are grass-fed, it is highly likely they will be antibiotic- and hormone-free. They may not be formally certified as organic, but that is typically irrelevant.

The organic certification is necessary only because most of us do not have the time to investigate the source of our food. When you purchase raw milk, it will typically be from a local farmer you will know and have an opportunity to question about their farming practices. This really is the ideal, and far healthier than relying on factory farming. The movement toward community-supported agriculture (CSA) is a powerful force that will help retain the value of the food supply and provide consumers with truly nutritional food that is not contaminated with pesticides and does not use GMO seeds.

If you have access to goat milk, it is even better than cow's milk, and the best animal milk of all is sheep milk. Because raw milk has normal flora bacteria in it, you can leave it outside the refrigerator for twelve to twenty-four hours, and it will turn into kefir—a fermented milk similar to yogurt but without all the added chemicals of the commercial product. I have used raw-milk kefir to help many of my sickest patients recover their health. Raw milk or raw-milk kefir is the only milk that your family should drink.

To sum up the content of this chapter, your body needs fluids, and the "liquid asset" it most craves is water. Water is crucial to the efficient functioning of your body. It keeps your body humming along the same way oil lubricates an engine to ensure its efficient operation.

Allow me (Dr. Lerner) to close this chapter with a powerful example of the difference good food and adequate water intake make in your body: As you probably know by now, poor health conditions are often due to poor food choices. When people start eating better foods, I have seen improvement—even total recovery—from nearly every illness known to man.

Joint problems, in particular, are often associated with the regular use of acid-causing foods. One of the most intriguing characters I've ever worked with was a man in his late thirties who was a former weight-lifting champion. He retired several years before seeing me due to severe arthritis in his knees and shoulders.

After learning about the acid-effects of certain staples in his diet like cheese, chocolate, coffee, tea, and processed red meat, he decided to consume them only on special occasions. Since none of the best doctors he had seen could help him, he really did not think simply changing his diet would help his arthritis. But he had nothing to lose, so he decided to try it.

The results were nothing short of a miracle. Within just a few weeks of eliminating these foods, adding good foods to his diet, and drinking an adequate amount of water, his joint pain had almost completely disappeared. The problems in his knees and shoulders would come back only when he put the acid foods back in his diet.

This man immediately went back to training and competing. Later that year, he won the championship again.

Now, be honest: after seeing such dramatic results, do you think that man was inclined to go back to his old way of eating and drinking? Not on your life! A lifestyle of health from wholesome eating and drinking pure water is your child's birthright also. It is our belief that you will see similar "miraculous" changes in your child's life as he embraces this new way of living.

So far you've learned about proper nutrition and the body's "liquid assets." But you may be wondering, What about vitamins and supplements? Where do they fit into my child's total health makeover?

We're so glad you asked—read on!

ARE SUPPLEMENTS ALL THEY'RE CRACKED UP TO BE?

9

If you listen to the message being sent by the vitamin and supplement industry, you'd think humans hardly existed prior to the advent of these convenient little pills. Their self-serving message is that the soils are depleted and it is "impossible" to get the nutrients we require from our soil. This might be true if you restricted your food choices to the typical grocery store. Well, folks, I simply don't buy it. We live in America, and we have many more options.

Biodynamic organic farms are currently producing vegetables that are likely to be among the healthiest vegetables ever grown in the history of the planet. These foods may not be the easiest to obtain in our current food distribution system, but the system is rapidly evolving to meet the demands of health-conscious consumers. The more educated and informed consumers like yourself demand this food from your local stores, the easier to find and less expensive these products will become. I have seen amazing progress in this area just in the past few years.

For the record, let me state that I believe you can obtain most of the nutrition you need from wholesome food. Americans have become far too dependent on pill-popping to take care of every need, even if that pill is a multivitamin.

There is little doubt that supplements can compensate for some of the damage we do to ourselves. However, my experience is that many, if not most, people use supplements to justify their poor food and lifestyle choices. About half the country takes nutritional supplements, and I suspect the percentage is considerably higher for others, especially people who classify themselves as "health conscious."

But if you stop to think about it, popping vitamins to ensure your body is "healthy" is like building a boat with rotten wood and using the best screws in the world to fasten it together. The boat may hold together, but it will still leak. The boards in the boat are like the macronutrients—the proteins, carbohydrates, and fats we consume. If we make poor choices at this foundational level, it really doesn't matter what type of screws we use—the boat won't float for very long.

Most vitamins serve as catalysts to reactions occurring in your body. There is no question that these catalysts are necessary, but good fuel (in the form of good food) is the best way to generate these reactions. A funny thing happens when you start out with good fuel (raw organic food): it has most of the vitamins and minerals you need packed right in there in the perfect balance—at no extra charge. Most of the new patients I see spend more than one hundred dollars a month on supplements, and a fair number of them spend more than five times that amount. Supplements will not fully compensate for not eating properly. Use food as your supplement, and you will be much healthier.

A Wise Greek Doctor

Hippocrates first popularized the "food as medicine" concept around twenty-five hundred years ago. Unfortunately, his advice fell into obscurity by the nineteenth century. The Industrial Revolution led to innovation in nearly all fields of study, and medicine was no exception. Think about how much health care has changed over the past century, for example. The first fifty years of the twentieth century saw the discovery of the essential elements and vitamins, particularly in the context of deficiency diseases. This led to the dubious practice of "enriching" processed foods to help people regain the health they lost when they abandoned whole foods. At the same time, the supplement industry—including everything from the infamous snake-oil remedies to modern-day multivitamins—found a lucrative market of eager (and sometimes gullible) consumers.

Unfortunately, the foundation of the "enrichment" movement is seriously flawed. The real solution to the epidemic of chronic degenerative disease in our culture is to establish a new and improved food distribution system that allows consumers to obtain whole unprocessed foods of high quality at a reasonable price. Only these types of foods contain the perfect nutrients, in the proper concentrations, that will reverse and treat disease. Relying on supplements to perform this miracle is idealistic fantasy.

An article in the *Journal of the American Dietetic Association* suggests that people frequently exceed safe nutrient levels when they take vitamin supplements. Similarly, an earlier study from the Harvard School of Public Health showed that popping a pill can't erase the health effects of a poor diet and a sedentary lifestyle. Higher intakes of folic acid, vitamin B_6, vitamin B_{12}, and vitamin D will benefit many people, the researchers found, and whole foods are the best source for these nutrients.[1]

I am a minimalist when it comes to supplements. Everyone has a unique metabolic and genetic variability, meaning the same supplement that helps one person with one disease could devastate the next person with the exact same disease. Multivitamins are particularly worrisome: If your body is sensitive to one component of the pill, then the supplement could end up promoting disease rather than health. The more nutrients in the pill, the greater the chances that your body may be sensitive, and the harder it is to determine the exact cause of the adverse reaction. For example, zinc has the potential to be toxic if too much is taken. Excess zinc can result in copper deficiency, which is associated with anemia.

According to one recent study, nearly two-thirds of chronically ill children use dietary supplements on a regular basis, and 30 percent use nonprescription supplements. Although some supplements can be beneficial, the study's researchers are concerned that the supplements' effects on children's growth and development are often unknown. Likewise, many doctors are often unaware that their patients are taking supplements, and in the case of chronically ill children, this increases the risk of drug-herb interactions.[2]

Having sounded the alarm regarding supplements, be aware that certain clinical conditions do warrant the use of nutrients and supplements as drug alternatives. Just remember to minimize the long-term use of supplements. If your child is healthy, he shouldn't be taking more than five supplements a day.

Fish Oil, Folic Acid, and Other Dietary Musts

Let me make it very clear that I do not classify fish oil as a supplement; I consider it a food alternative to fish. Our culture has managed to eliminate an entire class of food (fish) as a possible healthy option because of mercury pollution. Therefore, fish oil or krill oil is now the healthiest way to obtain the important omega-3 fatty acids that are absolutely essential for overall health.

The other supplement that is critical for individuals who choose not to eat animal protein is vitamin B_{12}. Few children are vegetarians, so hopefully this is not an issue for you, but it is a dietary approach that many in our culture follow. If your child does prefer a vegetarian lifestyle, be assured that the human body is quite forgiving, and healthy individuals can frequently tolerate this abuse for about seven years with liver reserves of B_{12}. But, after that time, the B_{12} deficiency frequently can cause irreversible brain damage.

Folic acid, a nutrient that helps prevent arteriosclerosis, heart disease, and neurological dysfunction, is best obtained by consuming large amounts of high-quality, uncooked, fresh vegetables. It is very difficult to overdo it on vegetables, especially if you listen to your body. Nearly everyone seems to benefit from eating as many vegetables as possible within the allowances of their metabolic type and body feedback.

The following table lists the folic acid content of some popular vegetables:

VEGETABLES (1/2 cup cooked unless otherwise indicated)	FOLATE CONTENT (mcg)
spinach	110
asparagus	88
collards	64
avocado, 1/2 raw	56
mustard greens	51
brussels sprouts	46
parsnips	45
beets	45
broccoli	38
endive, 1/2 cup raw	36
cauliflower	32
sweet potato	25
turnip greens	32
acorn squash	11

Vitamin E

This is one of the few supplements that I believe may be wise to use on a regular basis. However, recent studies have shown that the type of vitamin E most people use in their dietary supplements, alpha-tocopherol, may not be the ideal vitamin E supplement. It appears another form of vitamin E, gamma-tocopherol, the one mostly present in foods, is necessary to prevent cancers.

It appears that the alpha-tocopherol form of vitamin E has very few anti-cancer benefits. So if you are using vitamin E, please use a high-quality brand that has natural (not synthetic) mixed tocopherols, including gamma-tocopherol. Additionally, it appears that tocotrienols are vitamin E-like compounds that perform synergistically with vitamin E to further enhance its effect.

The Bottom Line

The bottom line on supplements is this: Don't be fooled by cheap substitutes. Whenever possible obtain your supplements from foods, not pills, and if you choose to do otherwise, beware of the unforeseen consequences. I encourage you to limit supplements in your child's diet and concentrate on feeding them from the earth's natural bounty of whole unprocessed foods.

Yes, there are some exceptions to this rule, but rarely does a person benefit from a shopping bag full of supplements. Here's a quick list of guidelines if you do decide to supplement your child's diet:

Lesson 1: Chromium May Help Sugar Cravings

Some people have found chromium helpful in controlling sugar cravings. However, it is far more likely that your child's sugar cravings are related to his or her overconsumption of carbohydrates.

Lesson 2: Avoid Iron in Your Child's Supplements

Although many children need iron, it is best not to get it from the inorganic forms present in most supplements. Additionally, it is important to understand that iron can be quite toxic, especially in the form present in most supplements. Accidental iron overdose from children consuming multivitamins with iron is a daily cause of death of children across the U.S. This is most tragic because if the iron in the supplement was carbonyl iron rather than ferrous sulfate, none of the children would die from the overdose.

Nearly all adult men and most menopausal women should avoid taking any iron supplements, as it is a major cause of heart disease and cancer. However, most children have greater iron needs than adults. Red meat is the best source of iron, so unless your child refuses to eat red meat, it might be best to avoid a multivitamin with iron in it.

Lesson 3: Carefully Evaluate Your Child's Need for a Multivitamin

Eating a healthy diet generally negates the need for a multiple vitamin, but you may want your child to take a multivitamin until he makes substantial progress on the Total Health Program. There's no question supplements can compensate for some of the damage that people do to themselves. But as I said earlier, in my practice I've found that most people use them to justify their poor food choices. No matter what you spend or what dosage you take, there is no substitute for proper eating. My biggest concern is that parents may be using supplements as a replacement for proper nutrition, which is the key to fighting so many chronic conditions.

Lesson 4: Make Sure Your Child Gets Enough Vitamin D

One of the many functions of vitamin D is to maintain normal blood levels of calcium and phosphorus in the body. Vitamin D is technically classified as a fat-soluble vitamin, but that really isn't accurate. Vitamin D isn't a vitamin at all but a prohormone. It is designed to be made from sunlight striking the cholesterol in your skin, which converts the cholesterol to vitamin D. You were never designed to take vitamin D pills. This is why even expert conventional pediatricians advise their breast-feeding patients to supplement their infants with vitamin D in the winter months as it is the only "vitamin" not present in human breast milk. That is because infants were designed to make it for themselves by being exposed to adequate sunshine on their bare skin.

During the summer months, your child will likely get enough vitamin D if he is spending enough time outside every day and you haven't slathered his skin with toxic and unnecessary sunscreen that completely shuts down the skin's ability to produce vitamin D. Encourage your child to participate in outdoor activities. It will be important to carefully monitor him in the early part of the season to avoid sunburn.

However, you can prevent sunburn by monitoring the time of day your child goes outdoors, the amount of time she is outside, and the use of protective clothing. As the season progresses, she should be able to tolerate longer and longer times outdoors without problems unless she is very fair-skinned.

Vitamin D deficiency is the most common vitamin deficiency in the country. If, for whatever reason, you or your child simply cannot get enough sun exposure, then it would be wise to consider supplementing your child's diet with cod-liver oil, which is high in vitamin D, vitamin A, and highly beneficial omega-3 fats. Vitamin A actually helps to limit vitamin D toxicity. Be aware, though, that cod-liver oil can vary greatly in quality; I have researched multiple brands and found Carlson's to be one of the best. If you can't find it in your local health-food store, for your convenience it is available on my Web site.

Lesson 5: Smell Your Vitamins

Vitamins may have a pungent odor to start with, but if that odor turns highly objectionable or causes you to be nausiated after swallowing them, consider this to be a giant clue. Listen to your body and stop taking that supplement. This is your body's way of signaling that something in the formulation is making your health worse.

If your child is on many supplements, you can get some help organizing them in a small fishing tackle box (available at most sporting goods stores). This is also a great way to transport the supplements when you travel.

Why You Should Consider "Going Organic"

Due to a growing demand for whole foods, many supermarkets today are adding organic food sections. Although the sale of organic food accounts for just 2.4 percent of the overall food industry, it has been growing at least 15 percent a year for the last ten years. Currently valued at $14 billion, the organic food business is expected to increase to $23 billion over the next three years. Even Wal-Mart plans on selling organic food.[3]

While the decision to purchase organic food versus conventionally grown food is a personal one, you may wonder: is organic food really better? Let me answer that question with an unequivocal yes. Organic farming differs from conventional farming in the methods used to grow crops. Traditional farmers apply chemical fertilizers to the soil to grow their crops, whereas organic farmers feed and build soil with natural fertilizer. Traditional farmers use insecticides to eradicate insects and disease, while organic farmers use natural methods such as insect predators and barriers to accomplish the same result organically. Traditional farmers control weed growth by applying synthetic herbicides, but organic farmers use crop rotation, tillage, hand weeding, cover crops, and mulches to control weeds.

As a result of all those chemicals, conventionally grown food is often tainted with chemical residues, which can be harmful to humans. The food industry entertains heated debates over what constitutes "safe" levels of these residues, but experts advise consumers to use caution. The Environmental Protection Agency (EPA) considers 60 percent of herbicides, 90 percent of fungicides, and 30 percent of insecticides to be carcinogenic.[4]

Pesticides can have many negative influences on health, including neurotoxicity, disruption of the endocrine system, carcinogenicity, and immune system suppression. Pesticide exposure may also affect male reproductive function and has been linked to miscarriages in women.

Pesticide contamination is not the only worry. Conventional produce typically has fewer nutrients than organic produce. Studies have found organic produce to contain significantly higher levels (up to 83 percent) of nutrients such as vitamin C, iron, magnesium, and phosphorus, and significantly fewer nitrates (a toxin).[5]

The results are in: organic foods are clearly superior to nonorganic foods. Yet many people who learn the truth about conventionally grown produce make the polar-opposite mistake of not eating any vegetables at all. They either cannot afford organic vegetables or have a hard time finding them. However, *please understand that it is better to eat nonorganic vegetables than to eat no vegetables at all.*

Also realize that fresh nonorganic vegetables are still better than wilted and rotten organic vegetables—sometimes the only ones available in smaller organic produce stands. Many highly perishable nutrients found in organic foods degrade with time and exposure to air and ultraviolet radiation. If the organic vegetables are seriously damaged, buy fresh, undamaged nonorganic vegetables instead.

It is my hope that the demand for organic food will drive a decrease in market prices, making this wholesome alternative available to the average consumer. If you must buy conventional produce, thoroughly wash all fruits and vegetables, although all pesticide residues cannot be removed by washing. You can also remove the outer layer of leaves or peel vegetables if possible. Another alternative is to grow your own vegetables, although this takes space, time, and climate considerations.

Another option is to buy organic produce selectively, as certain foods tend to have higher or lower amounts of pesticides. The following foods tend to have the highest levels of pesticides:[6]

FRUITS	VEGETABLES
1. peaches	1. spinach
2. apples	2. bell peppers
3. strawberries	3. celery
4. nectarines	4. potatoes
5. pears	5. hot peppers
6. cherries	
7. red raspberries	
8. imported grapes	

These foods tend to be lower in pesticide levels:[7]

FRUITS	VEGETABLES
1. pineapples	1. cauliflower
2. plantains	2. brussels sprouts
3. mangoes	3. asparagus
4. bananas	4. radishes
5. watermelon	5. broccoli
6. plums	6. onions
7. kiwi fruit	7. okra
8. blueberries	8. cabbage
9. papaya	9. eggplant
10. grapefruit	
11. avocado	

So far, we've covered nutritional changes that will help put your child on the path to true wellness. We've discussed the need for staying hydrated through adequate water intake, and which supplements are necessary for good health. At this point you may be wondering, "Okay, but how do I take all this information and make it work in my kid's life?" That's a big question that deserves a detailed answer. In the next chapter we'll take a look at steps you and your child can take to make healthy changes that "stick."

DR. BEN'S 5 QUESTIONS TO ASK
WHEN IT COMES TO SUPPLEMENTATION

1. SUFFICIENT: Am I taking a *sufficient* amount of nutrients needed to supplement (vitamins, minerals, amino acids, and fatty acids) in order to be well?
2. DEFICIENT: Is there some nutrient in particular that my body is *deficient* in?
3. ABSORPTION: Is my digestive system capable of normal *absorption* of the nutrients I'm taking?
4. QUALITY: Are the supplements and foods I'm using of the quality capable of being absorbed?
5. SAFETY: Am I possibly causing harm to myself due to the amounts, types, or poor quality of supplements I'm using?

For most, supplementation is incredibly ineffective. Commonly, people take the least expensive supplements they can find and load up on the products they've heard from the media, friends, or family were good for them or their children. With unneeded, poor-quality supplements, you might as well throw them directly into the toilet and skip the middleman.

Another method that's equally ineffective and even harmful is taking "This" for "That." If you're having an issue or concern, or a "This," you take supplements that are supposed to be good for "That."

The safest, most effective way to supplement is through a licensed health care professional who has been trained in this area and who can make an experienced assumption as to what you need. In our clinics we even do certain blood and urine tests to determine specifically what types and amounts of supplements you need to take in order to restore or maintain proper nutrient levels.

MAKING CHANGES
THAT STICK

Sticking to a brand-new way of eating is difficult for most people and nearly impossible for others. You may already be thinking, *Yep, you can include my child in that last category—I've tried everything,* but before you see the glass perpetually half-empty and give up, read the following "Seven Steps for Making Changes That Stick." These guidelines hold the key to positive, lasting changes in your child's life. Before we show you how to make these changes, however, here's a little background in what led to my (Dr. Lerner's) creation of these Seven Steps.

Early in my practice, as I worked with overweight people and encouraged them to eat better, I made a rather sobering observation: the average person would fail miserably. I gave my clients a detailed program for change, yet most of them not only did *not* lose weight but gained several pounds after only one session! How's that for un-success? Even cancer and diabetes patients would not follow my strict nutritional recommendations. At best, clients would stick to the new diet for a few days or weeks.

Over time, I became aware that this hard-core method of nutritional change—expecting someone to throw out her bad diet and immediately adopt a healthier one—generally doesn't work. So I went back to the drawing board and came up with seven ways to ease into a new lifestyle. As a result of the Seven Steps, I have seen results with thousands of people who thought they would never be thin or healthy again. Most of them had failed on numerous occasions to eat better.

The Seven Steps are designed to reverse the process of poor eating habits and move your child toward new, healthy eating habits. By taking the gradual route, you and your child will find yourselves making better and better decisions over time. The results will be a healthy body and a normalized weight.

Seven Steps for Making Changes That Stick

Step One: Addition

Positive eating is a gradual process. Your child didn't suddenly walk when she was a newborn; first she learned to crawl and then to pull herself upright, and finally she took that first step. Once you learn how to walk, nobody has to remind you to put one foot in front of the other—it's as natural as breathing. Changing eating habits is much the same way. To be effective and permanent, change must come slowly.

The Addition step states that instead of eliminating the bad, first add the good. Suppose your goal is to get your child to stop having soda and a sugary Pop-Tart for breakfast. That is a worthy goal, but you can't just stop that behavior and start feeding them nothing but eggs and fruit. If you do, they will only want to quit the program—and maybe throw a tantrum in the process.

The Addition step has you add an apple to your child's cola and candy bar breakfast. Remember, with addition you do not take away—you add.

Most people are overfed but undernourished. For the average American child, this statement could be doubly true. Think about the leeway society gives children and the junk food we "let" them have to satisfy their sweet tooth. Many modern diets (perhaps even your own child's) literally contain very little or even no real food at all. Most of it is fast food, junk food, quick food, and refined food, full of calories but devoid of nutrition. By adding healthy foods, your child becomes not only fed but nourished as well.

Have you ever noticed that the minute you're told to give up something, you feel an instant attachment to it and only want it more? Because of this all-too-human tendency, there is no Elimination step anywhere in this list of guidelines. The idea of elimination creates negative thought patterns in the brain. Our bodies respond better to "positivity" than to negativity. Eliminating negative food items from an unhealthy diet is much more challenging than simply adding positive foods a little at a time.

To begin thinking positively, take the first step toward change that sticks—Addition. No, adding an apple won't negate the ill effects of consuming unwholesome foods, but it will add a significant level of nutritional value to an otherwise entirely nutrition-free meal.

Over time the body will react so positively to these little additions that it will begin to crave healthier items as opposed to unhealthy ones. Gradually, those nutritional items that were once merely additions should become the entire focus of the meal.

Step Two: Replacement

We are bombarded by tempting treats everywhere we go: pizza, ice cream, cookies, sodas, sugared cereal, fast food—the list is a long one. Our cravings for these foods turn into literal addictions and create a real dilemma when trying to make a new start in healthy eating. To help avoid caving in to these cravings, take the second step toward lasting change, Replacement.

To help you, here is a list of commonly craved foods and their replacement foods:

CRAVING/ADDICTION	REPLACEMENT FOOD
1. Pizza: store-bought or homemade	1. Whole-grain pizza with all-natural sauce and low-fat unrefined cheese
2. Ice cream	2. Nondairy, low-fat alternative (e.g., Rice Dream)
3. Sugary, refined cereal	3. One of the many health-food, whole grain cereals with rice or almond milk
4. Sugar	4. Raw honey, fresh fruit juice, unrefined maple syrup, molasses, brown rice syrup
5. Salt, MSG	5. Healthy spices and condiments
6. Rich desserts	6. Whole grain, nondairy, chemical-free, low-fat, or raw-honey-sweetened or fruit-sweetened treats
7. Fast-food burger	7. Grass-fed organic homemade all-beef burger, organic turkey burger
8. Cheese	8. Raw organic cheese and nondairy cheese-like rice cheese

Many junk foods contain harmful ingredients such as preservatives, additives, MSG, and dangerous trans-fats. The good news is that today's health-food and grocery stores offer a variety of substitutes you can buy or make that are similar in form, satisfaction, and taste to these "addiction" foods.

To phase out unhealthy foods that leave your child overfed but under-nourished, follow the Replacement step and begin replacing food items with more health-conscious substitutes. Using these guidelines, your child will soon feel more satisfied after eating and may even be able to eliminate the old food cravings.

Step Three: 10-Point Reduction

On a scale of 1 to 10, a craving of 10 will be hard to resist. But if you can get that same craving down to a 7 or an 8, you can control it some or most of the time. Obviously, the lower you drop your cravings, the more success you will have over them. The 10-point reduction step helps you reduce a food craving down below a level 10, giving you more power over your decisions to consume.

First, you must identify those foods that cause your child a level-10 craving. Let's say, for example, your son craves ice cream. The thought of ice cream's sweet flavor and cool, creamy texture revs up his taste buds every time you drive by Baskin Robbins. If, however, you fed your son some low-fat plain yogurt tossed with fresh strawberries and blueberries, the cool, creamy treat would mimic the craving-food he loves but offer a much-healthier alternative. While the fruit and yogurt may not be as satisfying as ice cream, the similarity between the two would bring your son's craving down from a 10 to a 7. He may still want the ice cream, but the reduction in craving intensity allows him to skip the ice cream much of the time (again, think gradual).

Step Four: Vacation Foods

This fourth rule on my list of guidelines is everyone's favorite. Since it often takes years to undo poor eating habits entirely, it stands to reason that it will likewise take time to permanently change or give up poor food choices in favor of healthy ones. The Vacation step was created as a way of making this process of change much less stressful.

Like my parents when I was growing up, many people are either on a diet or off a diet. The nutritional plan offered in this book, however, is not a diet in the normal sense of the word; it's a new way of eating. It is something your child will work on for the rest of his or her life. No matter how satisfying any work is, you need a break from it now and then, and this new way of eating is no different. The Vacation food step puts a food, a meal, or even a whole day of less-than-ideal food choices on the menu plan. The idea that "if you crave, you cave" is a myth. Rather than calling it "cheating" when you give in to a craving, occasionally eating poorly is actually part of my nutritional guidelines.

While occasionally you will take a spontaneous vacation, the best vacations are planned. Make the Vacation foods on your child's diet the same way—plan to let them consume the foods they love in small portions, once or twice a week.

Suppose your child craves chocolate-chip cookies. Well, if she eats chocolate-chip cookies every day, she is going to keep gaining weight and worse. However, if you invoke Step 4, you set a short-term goal for when your daughter *will* eat chocolate-chip cookies. You might say, "You may eat chocolate-chip cookies only on Wednesdays and Sundays." Then on Saturday, when she passes the cookie counter at the mall food court, she is able to resist the craving because she has another "vacation" day coming up soon.

Some cravings are so great they are difficult to control—any adult knows this—and children generally are less self-disciplined than adults. But by setting a short-term goal for your child, usually she can push herself over the hump and make it another day or two.

With the Vacation food rule, your child may be able to drop some really bad eating habits entirely. By putting off some of her eating vices, she may find she is able to go completely without them.

Another positive side effect of this rule is that by isolating her craving-foods to certain days, your child may find that she doesn't feel well after eating them. She may discover she has a food sensitivity to these Vacation foods that she never noticed until she all but stopped eating them.

Go ahead—let your child eat "bad" foods once in a while, but don't give up on the nutritional program outlined in this book. After a short vacation with her favorite foods, let her get back to work. Eventually, this step will help your child enjoy life even without the vacations.

Step Five: Food Dress-Up

Let's be honest. Initially, some of the healthier food choices outlined in this book may not seem appealing to your child. Wholesome foods tend to appear less tasty and fulfilling because of all the additives, sugars, salts, and fats that give less-healthy foods their flavor. The reality is that natural foods do possess good taste, but our taste buds have been dulled by all the flavorings and spices in processed food.

In order to make healthy food more palatable to your child's desensitized taste buds, use the Food Dress-Up step.

For instance, unrefined oatmeal is a healthy breakfast choice generally free of all the toxic foodstuffs that dilute and debilitate other breakfast foods, such as cereals and doughnuts and bagels. The challenge is that oatmeal by itself does not contain much flavor, and preparing it with things like pasteurized sugar or dried fruit will negate some of its positive benefits. Plain old oatmeal and hot water can become a real chore for most people—your child is probably no exception. Even hot oatmeal and honey gets old after a while. To make this nutritious breakfast more appetizing, simply prepare "cool oatmeal."

Cool oatmeal is your standard oatmeal with different healthy items added to dress it up. Adding fresh fruits, almond or rice milk, sunflower seeds or cinnamon, granola, or healthy cereals will dress up the oats and make them more attractive and fun to eat without causing too much mischief inside your child's body. Dressing up wholesome foods is one way to avoid falling back into the Fruity Pebbles and Danish routine.

However, please understand that oatmeal is a grain, and if your child is suffering from severe obesity, even this relatively healthy grain could limit weight loss. It may be a food that you need to put on hold temporarily until you are able to get a good hold on the weight loss.

With this long-range goal of dressing up meals with healthy alternatives, proper nutrition can be achieved more realistically than by simply eliminating or giving up unhealthy foods altogether.

Step Six: Stay Full

Food choices are triggered by hunger. When hunger signals reach a certain threshold, it is nearly impossible to make healthy eating choices. That is why the Stay-Full step states that the way to achieve proper nutrition is to avoid getting too hungry.

Make sure your child consumes regular, healthy meals at appropriate times of the day. This will help him achieve a proper balance of staying nourished while also staying satisfied. On the other hand, skipping meals and going hungry lead to a practice of becoming "starved" and create the need for eating anything within reach to satiate the inevitable hunger pangs.

Unfortunately, when a person hits starvation mode, the most satisfying and often most available foods are those heavily refined, fast, or fried foods that are full of unhealthy fats and, often, sugar. To help your child avoid consuming such "junk" foods, make sure she stays full throughout the day with good, wholesome food.

Step Seven: Multiple Feedings

To achieve the Stay-Full step, it helps to also follow the Multiple-Feedings step. This last theory of proper nutrition states that smaller, lighter, healthier meals should be consumed throughout the day to avoid the intense hunger associated with weight loss. In a sense, you want your child to "graze" throughout the day rather than gorge at two or three large meals.

Your body is better equipped to process small amounts of food every few hours than to digest large meals spaced apart. Large amounts of food cause loss of energy, digestive dysfunction, and fat storage—the very thing your child is trying to fight. Going long periods of time between meals also slows down metabolism, making your child even less likely to burn those excessive calories.

Multiple small- to medium-sized feedings take less energy to digest, burn well, and speed up metabolism. To achieve ultimate results on the Beginner Nutritional Plan, make sure your child eats four to six times a day.

Lifestyle: Turning Choices into Changes

Along with Dr. Lerner's Seven Steps for Making Changes That Stick, we would like to share with you several basic lifestyle changes that are key to your child's success on the Total Health Program. Some of them overlap the rules but also provide new insights. Although most of these changes are common sense, it helps to outline them here so that you have a blueprint for success as you start your child down the path to optimal wellness.

Lifestyle Change 1: Teach Your Child to Control His Eating Habits (Where Age-Appropriate)

Vary your child's foods. Avoid serving your child the same foods every day of the week, namely to stave off the boredom factor. The goal is for him to enjoy the wholesome new foods you are introducing into his diet.

Have your child eat every few hours. The large amounts of grains and sugars popular in most diets cause us to have high levels of insulin circulating in our blood. When you stop or greatly reduce your grain intake, your body will take several days to lower insulin levels. In the meantime, the high insulin levels may cause symptoms such as dizziness, confusion, headaches, and an overall ill feeling. If your child eats every two hours for the first few days of her transition, she will be able to avoid this temporary side effect. Make sure she eats some protein, such as an egg, or a piece of chicken, turkey, or fish, along with a vegetable such as celery, cucumber, or red pepper. This will help prevent hypoglycemia and stabilize her blood sugar.

Encourage your child to eat more often during the day, rather than less often. Even after his system has adjusted, it will be wise to eat four to six meals a day. Eating more frequently normalizes cholesterol levels and also helps the adrenal glands better regulate cortisol levels. Cortisol levels regulate many of the body's other hormones, either directly or indirectly. When the adrenals are impaired, they can cause disruption in many other hormone systems.

Lifestyle Change 2: Make Sure Your Child Always Gets a Good Night's Sleep

One of the most important ingredients to a good night's sleep is to sleep in complete darkness. Any small amount of light in the room can potentially disrupt your child's delicately balanced biorhythms. This can impair her pineal gland's production of melatonin and serotonin. A simple, inexpensive strategy to block the light coming through the window is to obtain a large cardboard box and cut it to the size of the window. This works quite well but is not as cosmetically elegant as blackout shades or drapes.

If your child feels afraid in total darkness, it will be important to work with a therapist to quickly resolve this phobia.

In addition to darkness, I suggest these strategies for your child:

- Get between six and eight hours of sleep every night, and even more for very young children.

- Avoid watching TV immediately before bed—the stimulation may keep him awake; and even more importantly, take the TV out of the bedroom.

- Avoid using loud alarm clocks. There is a product called a dawn simulator that uses light to gently wake one up. You can find more information about these on my Web site or through a general Internet search.

- Keep the temperature in the bedroom lower than 70 degrees Fahrenheit.

- Get to bed as early as possible. Your body, particularly your adrenals, do a majority of their recharging or recovering between the hours of 11:00 p.m. and 1:00 a.m. If you are awake, this repair simply can't occur.

Lifestyle Change 3: Have Your Child Start Exercising, Especially if He Needs to Lose Weight

Dr. Lerner will go into more detail about exercise in later chapters, but it is quite clear that if your child struggles with weight issues, daily exercise is an effective tool to help. A child who needs to lose weight should gradually increase his daily exercise time to sixty minutes if at all possible. He may want to combine several shorter exercise periods to reach his daily sixty minutes. In the exercise portion of this book, we'll show you how to incorporate fun into your child's daily movements so he doesn't feel like he's exercising.

The synergy between diet and exercise is quite remarkable. And remember that exercise can take just about any shape or form that gets the body moving. One caveat: while swimming is one of the best exercises on the planet, if your child's only option is swimming in a chlorinated pool, I strongly advise considering other options. He will absorb more chlorine by swimming in a chlorinated pool than he would by drinking tap water for one week.

Swimming in a lake, ocean, or other natural water body is recommended (of course, always supervise your children when they're in the water). An ocean would be ideal and would actually be far healthier than a freshwater lake or river, as the salt helps kill certain bacteria on the body surface. If you have your own swimming pool, you can use products that contain peroxide (not bromine) as an alternative to chlorine. A product called Baquacil, available at most pool stores, uses this safe alternative to chlorine.

Lifestyle Change 4: Minimize Your Child's Use of Medications

Under your doctor's supervision, eliminate the unnecessary use of drugs from your child's regimen, and seek safe and effective alternatives when possible. Antibiotics are especially troublesome, as they destroy beneficial bacteria in your child's intestine.

You can review my Web site for many helpful strategies to wean your child off any medications. It is very rare that any child needs to be on a drug. There are nearly always effective natural alternatives. If the information on my Web site is not helpful, please be sure to identify a healthcare practitioner who is skilled in natural therapies to help you to carefully wean your child off any medicines they may be on.

DR. MERCOLA'S GUIDE TO A GOOD NIGHT'S SLEEP

Sleep deprivation will sap you of energy like almost nothing else. Children, especially, need their sleep—and lots of it. If your child is having sleep problems, including trouble falling asleep, waking up too often, or not feeling well rested when they wake up in the morning, try the following techniques:

- Have your child listen to white-noise or relaxation CDs. Some people find the sound of white noise or nature sounds, such as the ocean or forest, to be soothing for sleep. Young children may especially feel comforted by the sounds of nature as they drift off to sleep.

- Avoid letting your child have snacks before bed, particularly grains and sugars, which raise blood sugar and inhibit sleep. During the night, when blood sugar drops too low (hypoglycemia), your child might wake up and not be able to fall back asleep.

- As we mentioned earlier, your child should sleep in absolute, complete, pitch darkness. Any small amount of light in the room can potentially disrupt your delicately balanced biorhythms, which can impair your pineal gland's production of melatonin and serotonin.

- No TV right before bed. Even better, get the TV out of the house completely. It is too stimulating to the brain, and it will take your child longer to fall asleep. Watching television is also disruptive of pineal gland function for the same reason as above.

- Children should wear socks to bed anytime they have cold feet. The feet have the poorest circulation of the body parts and often feel cold before the rest of the body.

- Read something spiritual or religious together. For young children, bedtime Bible stories are ideal, but as your child grows allow her to read quietly on her own before lights out. This will help her to relax. Reading anything stimulating, such as a mystery or suspense novel, may have the opposite effect and lead to fitful sleep. In addition, if your child is engrossed in a page-turner book, she might wind up unintentionally reading for hours, instead of going to sleep.

- Avoid using loud alarm clocks in your child's room, which typically startle his body when he's in a deep state of sleep. Being awakened during this phase can actually harm his adrenals. We recommend he awake the way he was designed to, with natural sunlight. Until he's learned how to wake up, he can use a dawn alarm, an amazing device that wakes you up with light or sound (search for it on the Internet or visit www.mercola.com). If his body still requires additional sleep, he will sleep longer, which is one of its major benefits.

- Journal. If your child often lies in bed with her mind racing, encourage her to keep a journal and write down her thoughts before bed.

- Make sure your child gets to bed as early as possible. Our systems, particularly the adrenals, do a majority of their recovering between the hours of 11:00 p.m. and 1:00 a.m. In addition, the gallbladder dumps toxins during this same period. If your child is awake, the toxins back up into the liver and then secondarily back up into her entire system and cause further disruption of health. Prior to the widespread use of electricity, people went to bed shortly after sundown, as most animals do. I believe nature intended for us humans to go to sleep early.

- Check the bedroom for electromagnetic fields (EMFs). As strange as it sounds, EMFs can disrupt the pineal gland and the production of melatonin and serotonin, and cause other negative effects as well.

- Keep the temperature in the bedroom lower than 70 degrees Fahrenheit. Many people keep their homes, and particularly their bedrooms, too hot.

- Provide your child with a high-protein snack several hours before bed. This can provide the L-tryptophan needed to produce melatonin and serotonin. Also provide a small piece of fruit. This can help the tryptophan cross the blood-brain barrier.
- Avoid caffeine. A recent study showed that in some people, caffeine is not metabolized efficiently and leaves long-lasting effects in their bodies.[1] So an afternoon can of Coke will keep some people from falling asleep hours later. Also, some medications, particularly diet pills (which children should never be taking anyway), contain caffeine.
- Help your child lose weight. Being overweight can increase the risk of sleep apnea, which will prevent a restful night's sleep.
- Avoid serving foods your child is sensitive to. This is particularly true for dairy and wheat products, as they may cause sleep apnea, excess congestion, gastrointestinal upset, and gas, among other nighttime distresses.
- If your child avoids drinking any fluids within two hours of going to bed, this will reduce the likelihood of her needing to get up and go to the bathroom.
- Have your child take a hot bath, shower, or sauna before bed. When body temperature is raised in the late evening, it will fall at bedtime, facilitating sleep.
- Remove the clock from view. For fitful sleepers, constantly checking the time . . . 2:00 a.m. . . . 3:00 a.m. . . . 4:30 a.m. . . . only adds to their restlessness.
- Keep the bed for sleeping. If your child is used to watching TV or doing homework in bed, she may find it harder to relax and to think of bed as the place to sleep.
- Have your child's adrenals checked by a good natural-medicine clinician. Scientists have found that insomnia may be caused by adrenal stress.
- Get your child on a sleeping schedule. Every one of us should go to bed and wake up at the same times each day, even on the

weekends. This helps the body to get into a sleep rhythm and makes it easier to fall asleep and get up in the morning.

- Make sure your child gets daily exercise. Exercising for at least thirty minutes every day helps ensure a good night's sleep. However, don't let him exercise too close to bedtime or the adrenaline may keep him awake. Try having him exercise in the morning, afternoon, or early evening instead.

Dr. Ben's Guide to a BIG Brain

In the age of the brain, scientists are becoming increasingly concerned that we may be raising kids who can't use theirs. Of the many potential casualties related to today's high-tech, fast-food, fast-paced world, the inability of tomorrow's children to think may be at the top of the list.

Research over the last decade has revealed to us that thought and behavior in children and the relative size and weight of their brain are not something they're simply born with but something that's created or developed after birth. There's an intriguing term called *neuroplasticity* that essentially means our brains' neurological tissues are like formable plastic being molded, grown, and developed from birth through old age. This makes an allotment for two different scenarios:

1. You can develop a small, light, inefficient brain.
2. You can develop a huge, heavy, super-smart brain.

The power of neuroplasticity even works for the elderly concerned with or suffering from Alzheimer's. There's always something that can be done to change or improve brain function—for better or worse.

In the war between nature and nurture, the nurture side has been winning more and more battles. At the very least, we now know it's nature *and* nurture. We're presently aware of the fact that genetics doesn't necessarily determine outcomes. The physical, mental, and emotional environment we're exposed to—how we treat our body and what we feed it—have as much or more to say about how smart, happy, and healthy we are as our DNA.

Change what a child does with his/her brain, and you change the brain physically—as well as changing the child's future. This applies to IQ as well as nonintellectual intelligence—how a child succeeds and functions physically, socially, and emotionally in the world.

Keys to Building a Big Brain

- Lifestyle: A diet low in refined carbohydrates with adequate nutrients, extreme caution in the use of medication, adult companionship, the stimulation of active play, toys, books, and games, and limiting toxic foods and drinks.

- Parental involvement: Talk, listen, pay attention, and show children how to work through problems.

- Experience and adventure: Music, dance, walks in nature, art, pottery, caring for pets, and reading stories.

- Exercise: Brain development is also closely tied to motor systems and spinal health. Sometimes recess—playing kickball, climbing on the jungle gym—or a trip to the chiropractor does more for intellectual development than another page of math or history.

Keys to a Light Brain

- Lifestyle: Academic insensitivity, spinal or cranial injuries, medications, toxins, poor models from TV, movies, and video games.

- Technology: Overuse of technology devices acts as a nonhuman surrogate and takes time away from the most important needs children have for learning—social interaction, real-life experience, and creativity.

- Inactivity: Kids being forced to be attentive and grind out another math lesson while experiencing little time for activities may kick back with inattentiveness. This is normal and not a disorder of any kind. As doctors, we're concerned with the overdiagnosing of ADHD and hyperactivity, video addiction starting in toddlers and babies, the effects of stress and violent games on brain chemicals, and the fact that although society stresses the importance of mental function, it continues to feed our children toxic substances.

As the title of this chapter implies, the only real change is *change that sticks.* Adopting a little-at-a-time approach will help both you and your child experience success in the quest for wellness. But remember, good nutrition is only part of the solution.

GET MOVING!

11

Until now, we've focused on the nutritional changes necessary to start your child on the path to wellness and optimal weight. But that is only half the prescription for attaining optimal wellness. The other half is exercise. The body was built to move. All the vital parts that keep the body alive, including the heart, lungs, spinal cord, muscles, arteries, and so forth, require that you move on a consistent basis.

Regularly participating in sustained periods of movement positively and healthfully affects all parts and processes of your child's body. On the other hand, lack of movement leads to debilitation and, ultimately, lack of survival. In a very real sense, exercise may be the most important part of taking care of the body. Everyone eats, but other than using the jaw muscles for chewing, most people do not use their muscles on a regular basis. While nutrition is important, how often your child moves his body may be even more important than how often he eats.

Americans' love affair with the television and other trappings of the sedentary life has come at a high price, paid in the form of continual weight gain. The average weight of a ten-year-old has increased by about eleven pounds in the last forty years.[1] But keep in mind, that's only *average.* For many children, perhaps even your own, the scale has tipped way too far to the right—sometimes by as much as one hundred pounds.

To help move your child into the health and fitness zone, you must start by conquering EDS—exercise deficiency syndrome. Doing so will require shutting off the television and urging your child to get moving, and into the moving zone.

Most people don't appreciate how powerful exercise is; even many doctors fail to recognize the potency of this natural form of weight (and insulin) management. Like a prescription drug, however, if you don't use exercise in the right dose, it will not work.

Did you know that exercise alone is one of the most powerful healing agents we have in the treatment of type 2 diabetes? Unlike typical commercial drugs, exercise can actually cause a diabetic to go into permanent remission. In fact, with the added amount of preservatives, fat, additives, sugar, and other contaminants in our modern, processed food, physical fitness is even more essential than ever to avoid storing all that extra fat and eliminating all the sugar and poisons from the body. If your child is a "couch potato," over time that inactivity will cause him to live a shorter life, age faster, and grow larger. Seen in this light, exercise becomes nonnegotiable in the quest for wellness.

The Body-Brain Connection: Fit for Learning

We've all heard of the brain-body connection. But have you heard of the body-brain connection? While the brain controls and coordinates your fifty trillion cells, the brain still needs nutrients and stimulation coming from the body for its health and survival. Recently, studies in molecular biology have discovered how brain function and learning in children are affected by how we treat the body. These revolutionary findings have shown that the way brains learn is a profoundly physical and not a passive process.

John Medina, brain scientist and contributor to the work of the Talaris Research Institute, states, "Extensive research in the last two decades has shown that exercise can have strong positive effects on cognitive function, from improvements in pattern matching and problem solving to generalized improvements in memory."[2-3] This is an amazing discovery. We've heard of "food for thought"; now we have "exercise for thought." So when kids exercise, they have a dramatically better chance to learn and develop the mental skills necessary to succeed and thrive in life.

Sadly, contrary to these discoveries on exercise, today's fast-food, high-definition, high-tech video-game world has resulted in an overdramatically sedentary life—in other words, kids hardly move anymore. As a result, brain development, particularly the development of cognitive function (the ability to process ideas, create, strategize, and plan) is being greatly diminished.

At any age, exercise has been found to have both beneficial short-term and long-term effects on behavior and brain function. In school-age children, rigorous exercise creates dramatic improvements in academic performance, overall health, and social interaction.[4]

Among those who were reading disabled, a similar exercise program showed significant improvement in generalized literacy.[5]

In adults, exercise has consistently been determined to be a key variable for improved cognitive (brain) function.[6]

In old age, exercise is found to lower risks of general dementia and reduce the risk of Alzheimer's.[7] Even better, when combined with focused mental activities (puzzles, chess, etc.), exercise can slow down and in some cases reverse normal age-related memory loss as well as increase the speed of processing information.[8]

In Medina's investigation he stated, "A period of learning followed by intensive exercise dramatically improves key aspects of information processing when compared to non-exercised controls."[9] The beneficial aspects of exercise have been shown to act directly on the molecular machinery of the brain itself, and not just on more-generalized improvements in overall health.[10]

In the lab, exercise has had the following effects:

- Increased neuronal survival[11]

- Increased resistance to neural damage due to brain injury[12]

- Promoted overall brain vascularization[13]

- Stimulated generalized neurogenesis[14]

- Created stress-hormone resistance in vulnerable populations of brain cells[15]

In the books *Endangered Minds* and *Failure to Connect,* one of the country's best-known educational psychologists, Jane Healy, discusses the damaging effects of television on brain development in children. According to her, this is due to the fact that television is a passive activity that provides input into the brain but requires no physical movement. Essentially, if you're observing people, movies, games, or anything else you watch on TV and computer screens, but you're not physically engaging in these activities yourself, it is actually damaging to brain growth and function.

The American Academy of Pediatricians delved deeper into the issue of TV and concluded that no children two years old or younger should ever watch television—period. Again, the issue: television puts information into the brain while bypassing the mechanical aspects of the cerebellum. The fact is that the brain works through physical motion.

Additionally, computer screens and television tubes affect brain wiring. Creative activities, social interaction, and games that require strategizing and planning help develop the complex mechanisms of cognitive function. Our high-tech computerized games and toys, along with TV, do the creating and strategizing for us, allow for little thinking, and remove what life is all about—interacting with other humans.

As a chiropractor who works with children, my entire career is based on correcting spinal imbalances that can slow normal movement throughout the spinal column. These imbalances can lead to wear and tear on the affected spinal vertebrae and the involved areas of the central nervous system—the command center for all function in the body.

Much of the nutrition (oxygen and glucose) the brain needs for survival and operation comes from the fluid inside the spinal column (cerebrospinal fluid). Through motion, the spinal column pumps this vital fluid to the brain to keep it well. A properly functioning spine, coupled with regular physical activity, allows this pump to optimally send the necessary nutrients into the brain—the "body-brain connection."

The bottom line: Inactivity, television, and the like (video and computer games) are the enemy. Exercise and chiropractic are the heroes. Maximum motion = maximum learning and brain health.

Health and Happiness (No Pain, No Pain)

Top three excuses for not exercising:

1. Takes too much time

2. Too boring

3. Too painful

For true health and happiness, you need to find routines you like that fit into your busy day, that create results, and that you and your kids enjoy. Stress, even if from something that benefits you like exercise, is still stress. A child playing for half an hour on the playground is having a good time while simultaneously getting thirty minutes of aerobic exercise and a leg and arm workout. She is happy, getting healthy, and while working out hard—she is not in pain. *No pain, no pain.* That's the type of exercise we're suggesting.

Movement and Weight Loss

Weight loss accomplishes two important goals at the same time: not only will your child weigh less, but he will also be healthier. Unhealthy foods, diet products, strange devices, drugs, supplements, or herbal "speed" may make your child lighter, but not healthier. The only consistent way to lose weight and gain muscle mass is to eat healthy foods and exercise your body . . . period.

Losing weight does not necessarily promote better health. For an obese child, improved function of the body's operating systems requires not only less weight but also less *fat.* A person's weight alone is not what causes him or her to develop poor health and be susceptible to disease; rather, the person's ratio of body fat to muscle is the real culprit.

Exercise increases the body's amount of real muscle while diminishing the amount of loosely packed muscle, or what we call "fat." Having too little lean-muscle mass compared to body fat is a trigger for all sorts of conditions and diseases. High body-fat-to-muscle ratios negatively affect organ function, hormone balances, immune control, brain activity, and blood chemistry. People with such inverted body fat/muscle ratios are also typically more sensitive to sugar and cholesterol.

THE "SKINNY" ON FAT VS. MUSCLE

- Fat tends to produce more fat.
- Muscle tends to produce more muscle.
- Fatty tissue burns few calories.
- Muscle tissue burns more calories.
- Fat makes you tired and lazy.
- Muscle pumps up your energy.
- Fat contributes to a poor self-image.
- Muscle boosts confidence and leads to a healthy self-image.
- Fat increases your risk of disease.
- Increased lean muscle mass lowers your risk of certain diseases.

Everyone is looking for a silver bullet, an easy way to lose weight. But only diet *plus* exercise will increase your child's muscle-to-body-fat ratio. The positive result? Your child will not only weigh less, he will have better overall health.

Overturning Exercise Deficiency

While many people believe they are exercising enough, a closer examination of their lifestyle reveals they are seriously "under-dosed." The major reason most people quit or simply refuse to move regularly for extended periods of time is that it looks too painful or boring—or past experience tells them that it truly is too painful or boring.

The Miracle of Movement

Exercise's most amazing reward is that from the moment your child starts, many of her health dysfunctions resulting from being out of shape will improve or return to normal. You may be shocked at how quickly the body responds to a little vigor in the daily routine (we hope you are!). Dramatic changes such as lowered blood pressure or balanced blood-sugar levels are not uncommon.

What Exercise Does for the Body

- Improves heart function
- Lowers blood pressure
- Reduces body fat
- Increases bone mass
- Decreases LDL cholesterol ("bad cholesterol")
- Raises HDL cholesterol ("good cholesterol")
- Elevates energy level
- Balances hormone production
- Contributes to restful sleep
- Increases stress tolerance
- Eliminates toxins
- Reduces depression
- Controls or prevents diabetes (blood-sugar issues)
- Decreases the risk of injury to muscles, joints, and spine

EXERCISE: SEPARATING FACT FROM FICTION

Exercise Fiction: Exercising hurts.

Exercise Fact: Healthy movement is comfortable to the body and helps to prevent and overcome pain, not cause pain.

Exercise Fiction: It takes hours to exercise.

Exercise Fact: The positive impact of exercise starts from the moment you begin to move. Results can be seen in exercise that lasts as little as ten to fifteen minutes.

Exercise Fiction: You have to exercise in a gym or with extensive home-exercise equipment.

Exercise Fact: You can exercise just about anywhere: your home, neighborhood, or backyard, with some simple dumbbell, hand, or leg weights. These are all you need for a full-body routine to reduce fat, build lean muscle mass, and improve the cardiovascular system.

The "Active Lifestyle" Mentality

To foster a lifestyle of physical activity, help your child find routines he likes that easily fit into his (and your) schedule. If his fitness program causes stress for you or him, takes too long, or doesn't give him a healthier body fast, neither of you will stick with it.

While a child fourteen to sixteen years of age can get into adult-level programs, depending on her physical maturity level, the recommendations we're making go beyond simple routines. The most important part of living right is to develop an "active lifestyle mentality" and not one spent simply hovering around electronics.

To adopt an active lifestyle, you must begin with an *active lifestyle mentality.* For example, you bypass that prime parking space in favor of an "active" choice—the spot farthest away. Taking the stairs rather than the elevator or escalator is another good mentality to have. You might even make it into a game with your kids, seeing who can find the "worst spot" or counting steps.

One of the best ways to help your child get active is to enroll her in a team sport, such as Little League baseball, soccer, basketball, football, or other organized physical activities. The emotional boost that comes from being part of a team will be almost as valuable to your child as the physical benefits. Team sports are consistent, requiring practice several times a week (sometimes every day), and have regular games to show off the kids' prowess. When parents get involved, imagine how much more enthusiastic a child will be.

One word of caution: if your child's current weight or level of conditioning is too much of a challenge to participate in a team sport—either due to lack of strength or flexibility, or because you're worried about cruel teasing—get her started on some other form of exercise first until she sheds enough pounds or gets physically strong enough to feel confident about joining.

Team sports really are a wonderful way to kill three important developmental birds with one stone: your child gets social, emotional, and physical benefits.

Weight lifting, calisthenics, and jogging are all great habits to develop in the teen years. While many do not begin to "work out" until they're out-of-shape adults, strength training should begin earlier.

It's important to make sure your teenager has access to a place he can work out at home, at school, and/or at a gym. And *yes,* this is something you can enforce and hold him accountable to doing. Just like any other positive habit you enforce, the workout habit will pay incredible dividends in your child's future.

Lifting weights should not begin until your kids are fourteen or older. Middle and late-elementary school-age children under fourteen should perform a regular calisthenics program including push-ups, jumping jacks, sit-ups, squat thrusts, and other everyday exercises (examples later in chapter). This type of program avoids undue joint pressure and can even be considered fun.

Energy In = More Energy Out

There's a universal rule about exercise that many people don't know—at least not until they try it for themselves. Simply put, the rule states this: when you exercise, you get more energy than you put out. Isn't that amazing? Imagine your child comes home from school, exhausted by a grueling day of testing, and flops on the couch to watch TV. Traditional thinking assumes that when the body is feeling lethargic, it needs rest, but just the opposite is true. A lethargic, listless body needs to expend energy in order to gain energy back, and then some.

All in the Family

When children see a parent or older sibling exercising—and actually enjoying a physical activity—they can't help but "catch the bug" too. This contagion factor is capable of turning the E word (Exercise) into a three-letter word that starts with F: Fun. The following activity suggestions will help you prime the pump and get you, and your child, moving!

Parks and Yards

Find out where your local parks are and make a point of visiting them at least once a week with your child. To a kid, a park is a huge playground, and that's exactly what it should be. Get out there and play catch with your son or daughter, initiate a game of tag, take a nature hike through a wooded area, bike along an activity trail, or volunteer to pick up trash in a conservation area. The family backyard is another great place for physical activity—be creative and think of the fun, physical activities you enjoyed as a kid. Chances are, if you enjoyed them, your kids will too. It's all part of the active-lifestyle mentality.

No More Couch Potatoes

Reaching for the remote should not cause a grunt! Nor should tying your shoes, putting on your socks, or combing your hair. Flexibility saves joints, promotes good posture, and prevents injury. Transform your family television time into a game of sorts, seeing who can do the most sit-ups, squats, girl push-ups, or jumping jacks during the commercial break. If you have two or more kids, encourage a little competition between them, but be sure to keep it fun. My kids have come to expect this commercial-break activity time, and sometimes they can't wait for the commercials so they can improve their activity score! When they see Mom and Dad doing jumping jacks too, imagine how that motivates them to participate.

Nonfood Rewards

Good behavior, improved grades, and athletic accomplishments are often rewarded with junk food. Find more-positive rewards. It's conceivable that an overachieving child could weigh three hundred pounds due to his success before he/she graduates college.

Also, don't forget to reward kids for their wise nutritional choices and how well they've stuck to their exercise. While many parents are always looking to point out mistakes, let's be even more willing to point out and reward good decisions.

Sports and Games

Depending on your child's age, he or she may enjoy playing tennis or racquetball with Dad or a vigorous game of Marco-Polo in the pool. Capture the Flag, Frisbee, and backyard soccer are other good options for family activities that get everyone's blood pumping. Here are some other fun physical activities to consider:

- Duck, Duck, Goose

- Kickball

- Balloon Volleyball (played over the living room couch)

- Balloon Soccer (played in a den or cleared living room area)

- Nerf sports

- Wiffle ball toss

- One-legged races

- Potato sack races

- Relays

- Keep balloon in the air

- Water polo

- Basketball

- Jump rope

- 4-Square

- Hopscotch

- Bungee lifting (safe for age thirteen and under; either stand on Bungee exercise tube and stretch for resistance training, or mount in a door)

- Isometrics—squeeze exercise ball between feet, knees

GET MOVING!

Remember, the more energy you and your child put out, the more you get back. Here's a quick breakdown of how many calories you burn per hour from these ordinary physical activities:

- Sitting — 60
- Standing — 80
- Making beds — 155
- Housework — 150–250
- Strolling — 210
- Raking leaves — 225
- Lawn mowing (power) — 250
- Lawn mowing (push) — 300–400
- Gardening — 300–450
- Walking — 300–450
- Biking — 500–600
- Badminton — 550
- Square dancing — 550
- Leisurely swimming — 260–750
- Briskly swimming — 360–850
- Doubles tennis — 360
- Singles tennis — 480
- Volleyball — 300
- Light calisthenics — 360
- Strenuous calisthenics — 600
- Softball — 280–400
- Golf — 40–360
- Jogging — 600–750
- Moderate running — 870–1020

- Sprinting 1150–1285
- Leisurely skating 420
- Fast skating 700
- Downhill skiing 500–600
- Cross-country skiing 560–1020
- Basketball 560–660
- Rowing machine 840

(As you can see, just moving around burns three to four times the calories you use while doing nothing.)

Create a Fun, Daily Exercise Program

The exercises listed below are not only effective, they're playtime as well. Many organizations now exist to develop learning and physical skills through movement routines like the ones that follow.

Kids playing on a playground are having a good time while simultaneously getting thirty minutes of aerobic and anaerobic exercise. They are happy, getting healthy, and not in pain. Exercise should *never* hurt.

Kids thrive on routine, and they also love it when their parents play with them. Find a half hour in their day when you can jointly do the following movements. Remember that a little movement, done consistently, adds up to a lot of calories spent and increased physical fitness, flexibility, and overall health—for both of you.

These movements don't require a lot of space, so find a place that suits your lifestyle and surroundings: a park or playground, the back porch, the backyard, your child's bedroom. Are your kids tied to the TV? No problem. You can even do these movements in front of the tube. Make a game of it and perform the various movements during their favorite half-hour TV show. Once the half-hour exercise program becomes "easy," graduate to a full hour of movement.

Keeping Kids Moving for Thirty to Sixty Minutes

Let's suppose you choose to do the following movements in a cleared space in your family room, while watching TV. Have a few simple exercise aids on hand, such as a hoola hoop, a stretchy (exercise) tube, and a midsize bouncy ball.

You might begin by saying, "Okay, Johnny, let's see how many different movements we can do before the end of the show. Here's the catch: Every time the program goes to a commercial, we have to add a piece of equipment to mix things up. We can do the hoola hoop during the commercials, or toss the ball back and forth, or do stretching exercises with a stretchy tube. When the TV program starts back, we will do our regular movements again."

Here are some movements to incorporate into your workout: march, fly, wiggle, twist, pause, spring, creep, dodge, spin, dig, swoop, waddle, twirl, shrug, punch, slither, sweep, clap, slide, leap, swing, crawl, jump, hop, roll.

For example, begin by marching in place for five minutes then add a shrugging motion to the movement (that one little addition will strengthen their shoulder muscles).

Next, you may want to change things up by switching to a twisting motion or a duck waddle. Use your imagination and keep it interesting. If your child is young, you might tell him to pretend he's a snake: "Show me how a snake slithers on the ground." Or let him pretend to be a frog instead and hop around the room.

Add Variety by Mixing It Up

You may want to change up the routine so your child doesn't get bored. For example, ask her to do the movements fast/slow, high/low/medium, zigzag/curvy/straight, forward/backward, alone/connected, right/left.

For older children, ask them to perform, say, fifty jumping jacks or push-ups during every commercial break, or get down on the floor with them and do as many sit-ups as you can before the TV program returns. During the TV program you could perform other traditional calisthenics, such as leg raises, doggie lifts (down on all fours), windmills (bend at the waist and twist while swinging arms from side to side), or heel raises. The movement possibilities are almost endless. The idea is to keep them moving and to have fun while doing the motions.

Musical Movements

Not every child will want to do the movements in front of the TV. Another fun option is to use music as a component of the movement routine. Have a stereo boom box nearby and start and stop the music to start and stop your child's motion. As in the game Musical Chairs, have your child perform one movement until the music stops and then freeze in place. When the music starts again, ask her to change motions. See how many different movements you can do together during a half hour of songs. You may want to choose eight three-minute songs for twenty-four minutes of one activity, then take a short break and switch to another activity.

When it comes to adding a movement routine to your child's life, use your ingenuity as a parent and your child's own creativity to create a program both of you will enjoy doing together. Making physical activity a daily part of your life will help you and your child naturally adopt the active-lifestyle mentality.

Quick Sets for Teens

To get your teens working their maturing muscles quickly and effectively, try these quick sets. They can work with dumbbells or calisthenics and get through powerful workouts in only minutes.

Teens can work each body part one to two times/week and do calisthenics four to five days/week.

Two Quick-Set Categories:

1. Decline Set (with dumbbells)

- Pick one exercise and do it for 8–12 repetitions until failure (example: do as many bicep curls as you can).

- Rest 5–6 seconds.

- Lower the weight 5–20 pounds and do the exercise again for 6–8 repetitions until failure.

- Rest 5–6 seconds.

- Lower the weight 5–20 pounds again and do another 6–8 repetitions until failure.

When done, you've completely worked out that body part and can move on to another body part. For more ambitious exercisers, you can do more than one exercise for a body part.

2. Pause Set (done with weights or calisthenics)

- Pick one exercise and do it for 8–12 repetitions or until failure as with push-ups or sit-ups.

- Rest 5–6 seconds.

- Using the same weight or doing the same exercise, do the exercise again until failure.

- Rest 5–6 seconds

- Repeat this process until you cannot do the exercise for more than 1–2 repetitions.

Example:

- Do push-ups until you can't do any more (e.g., 15 repetitions).

- Rest 5–6 seconds.

- Do push-ups again until you can't do any more (e.g., can do 10 more).

- Rest 5–6 seconds.

- Do push-ups again until you can't do any more (e.g., can do 5 more).

- Do push-ups again until you can't do any more (e.g., can do 2 more).

  You're now finished with push-ups.

For more information on "Quick Sets" see Dr. Ben's book *Body by God: The Owner's Manual for Maximized Living* and/or the Quick Set Video available at www.maximizedliving.com.

P.E. GETS BENCHED[16]

Physical-education experts say there's little accountability for P.E. teachers in most schools. They say the classes are often poorly run, and students don't spend much time in them anyway—even as American children grow fatter and more out of shape.

The Centers for Disease Control and Prevention reports that in 2003, only 28 percent of high school students nationwide attended a daily P.E. class, but 38 percent watched television for three hours or more each school night.

While 71 percent of the nation's freshmen were in P.E. at least one day a week—hardly enough to be effective, experts say—those numbers drop to 40 percent by the students' senior year.

National Association for Sport and Physical Education president Dolly Lambdin said the cuts in secondary schools and colleges intensify the problem that begins at a young age.

"Whatever belief we teach [children] in elementary school, middle school and high school, those beliefs will carry over in college," she said. "We can't continue the model we have to fix things later. It doesn't work on your car and it doesn't work on your body. Physical maintenance is the key."

In the next chapter, we include several activities and programs appropriate for very young children—toddlers and preschoolers. If you don't have a child this age, skip over to chapter 13.

MOVEMENT ACTIVITIES FOR TODDLERS AND PRESCHOOLERS

Early childhood is the age of exploration for kids—the world holds endless wonders and their minds soak up information like thirsty sponges. Remember how fascinating dandelions, fluffy white clouds, and even garden-variety bugs were when you were young? It's also a critical time for a child to discover the world around her. This occurs, with a little encouragement and participation by you, with physical activity as a regular part of her life.

For young children, all exercise should really be "play" rather than a heavy-duty regimen. All of the exercises in this chapter are designed with parent and child in mind and simulate activities children naturally do when they play alone or together.

Before we get into the exercises, let's take a brief look at how toddlers and preschoolers—ages two to five—see the world.

Physical

At this age, kids are usually slightly farsighted. They have some perception of height and width and are able to locate and identify body parts ("this is my nose, this is my elbow," etc.). At this point children have greater tactile perception in the upper body parts, and they have mastered the art of heel-to-toe walking.

By ages three and four, children have the ability to climb and descend from a ladder and can use their arms to balance on one foot. They can also stretch upward and maintain balance. Rhythmical skills are starting to develop. At this age, children are able to roll a ball by holding it at the side of the body. They have limited striking, catching, and throwing skills and demonstrate success in running, jumping upward and forward, hopping, and galloping.

Intellectual

By this age, children's reasoning skills become more obvious. They may rely on the shape or form of an object for identification rather than on color. However, they are able to differentiate between basic colors and shapes. They recognize the letters of the alphabet and are proficient at drawing vertical, horizontal, and circular lines. Other skills noted at this age are the ability to illustrate objects or pictures reflecting personal experiences, manipulating clay in rough 3-D forms, folding paper vertically and horizontally, exploring and experimenting with manipulatives, and understanding the difference between touch, feel, smell, and taste.

Emotional

The young child has a vivid imagination and often constructs imaginary play fantasies with imaginary plots. A fascination with adult roles shows up at this age, along with emotional extremes. Young children desire attention and praise and easily express feelings of likes and dislikes. They are very curious about the environment and show signs of self-confidence.

Social

Young children demonstrate cooperative play and the ability to interact with others to achieve a common goal. They are beginning to have some appreciation of their peers' viewpoints but share objects with reluctance. Aware of gender differences at this age, a child waits for his or her turn and enjoys peers who have similar play interests.

Creating a Movement Environment

Young children need the opportunity to perform movement activities in a safe, parent-supervised environment. You may want to invest in play structures like jungle gyms and so forth, but you don't need to go to this expense. Instead you can use simple (and inexpensive) objects such as jump ropes, hula hoops, balls, and beanbags to accomplish these exercises. The absence of a spacious "play-room" or home gym should not prevent any child from taking part in purpose-ful movement activities. The bottom line for young children is to make that purposeful movement fun.

Movement Activity: Cinderella/Johnny Appleseed

Let's suppose you choose a section of your den or screened porch for activity time. As you prepare to do these exercises, you could ask your daughter to imagine she is Cinderella, sweeping the kitchen while her stepsisters get ready for the ball. Do sweeping motions all around the room to carry the role-play out. If you have a son, let him pretend to be Johnny Appleseed, bending to plant apple seeds in the ground. See how many different apple trees you can plant together. The words "let's imagine . . ." alone are enough to spark any young child's enthusiasm. Other themes could include pretending to be Santa's elves or Snow White's seven dwarfs.

Developing an Understanding of Space

Turn your parent-child exercise time into an opportunity to teach him about the concepts of personal space and general space. Spatial-awareness activities also teach a child how to avoid fixed objects when moving at various speeds, how to move safely through obstacles, and how to move over different types of surfaces.

Movement Activity: Hatching Baby Dinosaur

Ask your child to pretend she is a baby dinosaur inside an egg. You might tell her, "Can you reach out and feel the shell around your body?" Let her exper-iment with different actions inside her "egg," such as the following:

- Move just one body part.
- Move two body parts at the same time.
- Reach both arms up high.
- Lie down in her egg.

- Curl up in a ball.

- Pretend the egg has hatched and push through the shell.

A CHILD'S UNDERSTANDING OF SPACE

Young children gradually learn about the different kinds of "space" that occupy their world: Personal Space and General Space. They learn that they can move within their own Personal Space as well as through General Space, interacting with the people and environment around them. Over time, they realize that movement can take place at different speeds—slow, moderate, fast—and several different directions: beside, forward, backward, sideways, upward, downward, straight, zigzag, circular, curved.

Movement Activity: Run, Run!

Ask your child to try the following activities while running across the yard or a cleared space in your home:

- Run with hands high in the air.

- Run while lifting his knees.

- Pump his arms as he runs.

- Run and stop at a high level.

- Run and stop at a low level.

Movement Activity: Hippity-Hop

Challenge your child to try these variations on hopping like a bunny:

- Hop up and down on one foot and then change to the other foot.

- Hop backward.

- Hop over a jump rope or a chalk line drawn on the floor.

Movement Activity: Galloping Pony

Encourage your child to transition from hopping to galloping like a horse:

- Gallop and pretend to hold the reins of a horse.
- Gallop alongside you or a playmate.
- Gallop backward.
- Gallop in a large circle.

Movement Activity: Skipping

- Skip while placing hands on hips.
- Skip while humming a song.
- Skip in a circle, a triangle shape, a square shape.
- Point her toe and skip in that direction.

Movement Activity: Boxes

Children love playing with boxes. Now you can make a physical activity out of "box play" by using a "Simon Says" format:

- See how quickly he can stand in front of the box, to one side of the box, and behind the box.
- Move away from the box, stop, and then move toward the box.
- Hide inside his box.
- Hop on one foot around the box.
- Skip around the box.

Movement Activity: Everyday Movements

Remind your child that we use specific movements to perform different tasks as we go about our daily routines. Challenge her to perform the following movements through make-believe:

- Dress for school.

- Put away her toys.

- Play with her pet dog or cat.

- Get ready for bed.

- Use a broom to sweep.

- Carry a bag of groceries.

- Stir a large bowl of pudding.

- Rake leaves into a pile.

- Push a lawn mower.

- Pull weeds with long roots.

- Use a shovel and dig a large hole.

TRAVELING ACTIONS

The most basic exercises we were all created to do is to move ourselves in a variety of ways from point A to point B. For children and adults, these kinds of natural movements are even better than modern exercise equipment. They take joints and muscles through a very natural range of motion, safely and effectively building them and preparing the body for taking on whatever life has in store for it.

• Crawling	• Jumping	• Leaping
• Hopping	• Tiptoeing	• Hiding
• Galloping	• Swimming	• Strutting
• Rolling	• Skating	• Marching
• Running	• Flying	• Waddling
• Sliding	• Pouncing	• Slithering

Movement Activity: Stretchy Man!

Show your child how different items can stretch, such as gum, elastic bands, or Silly Putty. Challenge him to stretch by doing the following:

- See how far he can stretch his body with arms outstretched (overhead).

- Stretch his ankles by standing on his toes.

- See if he can stretch only one side of his body.
- Try curling and stretching his toes.
- Stretch his arms and reach from side to side.
- Do a SUPER STRETCH!

Movement Activity: Alphabet Soup!

Explain that each letter in the alphabet can be used to create a movement word. Ask your child to perform these stretching movements:

- A is for Air. Can you take three big breaths of air?
- B is for Bouncing. Can you bounce like a rubber ball?
- C is for Curling. Can you curl your body into a round shape?
- D is for Dodging. Can you dodge to one side and then to the other side?
- E is for Exploring. Pretend to explore a long, dark cave.
- F is for Fun. Show me how your body moves when it is having fun.
- G is for Grip. Can you curl your fingers and make a tight fist?
- H is for Hug. Give yourself a great big hug.
- I is for Inflate. Let's pretend to blow up a giant balloon.
- J is for Jump. Try to jump upward and touch the ceiling.
- K is for Kick. Show me how you can kick an imaginary ball with your foot.
- L is for Lower. How slowly can you lower your body to the floor?

Movement Activity: The Ceiling Is Falling!

Encourage your child to stretch and push in the following ways:

- Let's make believe the ceiling is moving downward. Can you pretend to push it upward above your head?

- The wall in front of you is moving closer. Push it away from your body.

- Now the walls at your sides are moving closer. Stretch your arms and push them away from your body.

- Oh, no! The floor is shrinking. Can you stand on your tiptoes as this space shrinks in size?

- Now stretch as high as you can to keep our activity area very large.

The exercises found below are broken into specific age-groups—toddlers and preschoolers—and will help your child accomplish a variety of movements while having fun. Your involvement in these exercises will reinforce a positive attitude toward physical activity. Eventually your child will pick up the message: exercise is something to look forward to!

Toddlers

The following exercise games are designed specifically for very young children. You can start as early as your child is able to walk.

Heads, Knees, Toes

This game helps with identifying body parts, flexibility, and understanding the concepts of up, down, low, and high.

- Stand facing your child.

- Beginning slowly, call out the names of the three body parts that are in the title, asking your child to touch each part as he hears its name.

- Once your child is successful at this, reverse—and mix up—the order of body parts.

Also:

- Change the tempo at which you call out the body parts—sometimes slow and sometimes fast.

- Another possibility is to start out slowly and gradually get faster.

- When your child is ready, play Heads, Shoulders, Knees, and Toes. Later you can once again change the order of body parts and the pace at which you call them out.

Walk on Tippy-Toe

Walking on tiptoe uses the child's own body weight to develop strength. It also helps with balance.

- Show your child how to tiptoe.

- Ask her to do it with you.

- Tiptoe as long as your toddler stays interested.

Also:

- Play a piece of quiet music as you both tiptoe.

- Use imagery—for example, ask your child to pretend she's sneaking up on someone, or a kitty cat trying to catch a bird.

- Vary the way you move (straight, curving, and zigzagging) and directions (forward, backward, and sideways).

"Row, Row, Row Your Boat"

This game works on strength and flexibility, while also teaching about cause and effect.

- Sit facing your child with your legs apart and your child's legs straight out, between yours.

- Holding your child's hands, lean forward and encourage him to lean back as far as he can.

- Pull him gently back up to a sitting position. Repeat.

Also:

- Sing "Row, Row, Row Your Boat" as you gently rock back and forth.

- As your child becomes stronger, you can also lean backward yourself, causing him to lean forward.

Gallop-Go-Round

Show your child how to gallop (leading with one foot while the other plays catch-up). If you do this activity for long periods of time, it helps build up your child's heart health.

- Ask her to gallop behind you.

- Make a game of Follow the Leader, and take turns being the leader.

Also:

- If your child isn't yet ready to gallop, have her pretend to be a horse. She'll be galloping before you know it!

- Give your child a stick horse or a small, child-sized broom. This may make it more fun and help her learn to gallop.

- When your child knows how to gallop, have her try galloping with her other foot first.

More Ideas for Toddlers

- Follow the Leader: Play this fun game using all of the traveling skills your child has learned (walking, running, tiptoeing, jumping, etc.). Stop once in a while to do a stationary (in-place) skill, like stretching, bending, or twisting.

- Mother May I: Remember this game from your own childhood? The "Mother" stands several yards away and calls out a movement, and the game participants have to do that movement as they progress toward Mother. Motions include waddling like a duck, taking baby steps, giant steps, zigzag steps, sideways steps, frog leaps, bunny hops, etc. Let your toddler go through all the motions, and when she reaches you give her the chance to be the Mother.

- "Pop Goes the Weasel": Hum or sing this age-old favorite, asking your child to move around the room until the "pop," when he should jump into the air. Later you can ask him to jump and change directions when he hears the pop.

- Kangaroos: Invite your toddler to jump as though she were a kangaroo. Ask her to see how far she can jump each time.

Preschoolers

By the time they're preschoolers, children are able to do movement activities that involve multiple actions.

Heel Raises

Lifting and lowering the heels is a strength-training exercise even the youngest children can do. It also helps with balance.

- Stand facing your child.

- Hold hands.

- Slowly lift and lower your heels, encouraging your child to do the same thing at the same time.

Also:

- Pause each time you rise onto tiptoe, counting aloud to five.

- Instead of just raising your heels, you and your child can jump (two feet) or hop (one foot) lightly in place.

- Try all of these activities both slowly and quickly.

Beanbag Balance

When it comes to balancing activities, this is an all-time favorite for children.

- Place a beanbag or a small, soft toy on your child's head.

- Invite her to walk from one point in the room to another without dropping the beanbag.

- If she has to, she can hold on to it at first.

Also:

- Ask her to balance the beanbag as she walks both slowly and quickly, in different directions (forward, backward, or sideways), and in different pathways (straight, curving, and zigzagging).
- Invite her to try balancing the beanbag on other body parts, like a hand, shoulder, or elbow.

Jump the Creek

Jumping uses the child's own weight to build strength. If you do this for long periods of time, it can be good for the heart.

- Lay a jump rope in a straight line on the floor—or draw a line on the ground with chalk.
- Ask your child to pretend the line is a creek.
- Challenge him to jump from one side of the creek to the other.

Also:

- Be sure your child is landing with knees bent and heels coming all the way down to the floor.
- When he's ready, you can "widen the creek" by using two ropes, side by side, or a towel.

Mirror Image

This cooperative game is great for social/emotional development. And it means children have to do with their bodies what their eyes are seeing. This will help later with writing, among other things.

- Talk to your child about looking in the mirror.
- Stand facing your child, explaining that you want her to do exactly as you do—as if she were your reflection in the mirror.
- Begin making slow movements that you can do in place, like raising and lowering an arm, nodding your head, or clapping your hands. Take turns being the leader.

Also:

- To help your child be more flexible, do things like bending and straightening at the waist, stretching arms overhead, or slowly reaching for your toes (keeping knees slightly bent).
- To help with muscle strength, lift and lower the heels or do deep knee bends.
- To help with heart health, jog or jump in place, stopping occasionally to rest.

More Ideas for Preschoolers

- Bridges and Tunnels: Forming different kinds of bridges and tunnels with the body or body parts can help with both flexibility and muscle strength.
- Olympic Track Meet: Invite your child to pretend she's in a track meet at the Olympics. Can she pretend to jump hurdles, in addition to "running the track"?
- Simon Says: Play this excellent body-parts identification game without any elimination! To include fitness factors, have "Simon" issue challenges to jog or tiptoe in place, bend and stretch, or bend and straighten knees.
- Stone Statues: To get your child moving, put on a piece of up-tempo music and invite him to move while the music is playing and to freeze into a statue when you pause the music.

If you approach the exercises in this chapter as "playtime with Mommy or Daddy," your child will look forward to his daily romp—and maybe even beg for more. The desired outcome, of course, is he develops an early love for physical activity and associates it with positive mental reinforcements: Exercise = Fun!

TYING IT ALL TOGETHER 13

You've come this far, packed your brain full of information, and perhaps are feeling a bit overwhelmed right now. Relax. This section has been designed to help you pull everything together and make sense of the extraordinary changes you are about to make in your child's life.

Please remember that if you fail to plan, you are planning to fail, so we highly recommend you create a plan to adopt the program in "manageable bites"—for you and your child. As you start your child on the Beginner Nutritional Plan, refer to this book often, rereading the chapters that offer key points and food guidelines.

Keep It Simple

Here's a 1-2-3 plan for staying on track:

Month One

- Use the test in chapter 7 to get a basic idea of your child's metabolic type.

- Start cutting added sugars and processed grains from your child's diet.

- Start feeding your child more of the right vegetables for his carbohydrate needs.

- Start introducing healthy alternatives to your child's favorite foods.

- Start giving your child fish oil, vitamin E, and probiotic supplements daily; eliminate unnecessary supplements.

- Start watering down your child's juice, and introduce pure water into his diet.

- Aim for fifteen minutes of exercise three times a week to start.

Month Two

- Keep working toward any of the goals from the previous month.

- Wean your child off soda by gradually cutting him down to one glass a day.

- Increase your child's water intake daily.

- Make sure your child gets adequate sleep every night.

- Increase your child's exercise to thirty minutes three days a week.

Month Three

- Keep working toward any of the goals from the previous month.

- Cut all processed grains (anything but whole grains) from your child's diet.

- Continue to wean your child off soda; cut back to one glass every other day.

- Increase your child's exercise to thirty minutes fives days a week.

Month Four

- Keep working toward any of the goals from the previous month.

- Limit soda to one a week or eliminate altogether.

- Increase your child's exercise to thirty minutes every day of the week (eventually you will help her reach the ideal of sixty minutes daily).

Painting Solid Yellow Lines

If you have a full-time job, a family, and a desire to implement all the elements found in this book, you may feel like you need to become a black belt in time management. The truth is, there is always enough time to get the important things done. The problem is never the lack of time; the problem is lack of time *management.*

Our lives are complex. You probably have a lot of rows in your garden. Any row that is left unwatered and unattended is going to fail to flourish— or die altogether.

Let's count your lives:

1. Relationship life

2. Parent life—if you have more than one child, then there is more than one life here

3. School life (learning continues throughout your life, long after "school" is over)

4. Work life

5. Health and fitness life

6. Purpose and mission

Kids have a bunch of lives too, if you consider school, relationships, family, and extracurricular activities like sports, cheerleading, or music.

If you and/or your children have any chance of thriving in each of these areas, organization and planning are vital to making it work. We teach chunking or compartmentalizing your life or lives by a system called "Painting Solid Yellow Lines."

When you are driving, if there is a dotted yellow line, you can pass or cross over into the other lane. However, if there is a solid yellow line, you cannot (legally) pass and you cannot (legally) cross over. Others cannot pass or cross over either. If you paint solid yellow lines around each of your lives, other lives and activities cannot pass or cross over—and the activities in each of those lives stand a better chance of actually getting accomplished.

Solid Yellow Line Example for Adults

6:30–7:30 a.m.:

Family Life (assuming that you are married and/or have children).

7:30–11:00 a.m.:

Work Life. There is a solid yellow line drawn between Family Life and Work Life. You drive to the office, do your job with excellence, and focus from 7:30 a.m. to 11:00 a.m. At 11:00 a.m. another solid yellow line is drawn and you begin another life. Sometimes it's nap life—but it's still scheduled. Just like in kindergarten.

Each day has your separate lives. All other lives are strategically placed throughout the week so everything that needs to be accomplished is done *well.* Obviously, it doesn't always work out so perfectly. Sometimes a child interrupts during times designated for reading or an urgent issue pops up that needs to be handled. At those times, you have to practice flexibility. You do not want to become massively stressed when something or someone tries to get by you in the "no-passing lane."

If lives "cross over" into other lives, as they occasionally will, try to remember the admonition, "That's life." Work to get past the issues and try to get everyone and everything back in their lanes as quickly as possible before there is an accident!

Unfortunately, a few times a year there are some traumatic, stressful five-life pileups. But, by getting back to proper compartmentalization through the painting of solid yellow lines and proper delegation, you will usually manage to escape with only some minor damage.

Solid Yellow Line Example for Children

If a child has baseball, homework, piano lessons, and he loves to play video games, you allow a specific time or times for all of those during the week.

1. YELLOW LINES AROUND 4:00–5:30 p.m.

DAILY: SCHOOL LIFE

A. Schoolwork

B. Reading

C. Educational video

2. YELLOW LINES AROUND BASEBALL PRACTICE 3:00–4:00 p.m. M,W, FR

3. YELLOW LINES AROUND PIANO LESSONS 12:00–1:00 p.m. ON SATURDAYS

4. YELLOW LINES AROUND 5:00–6:00 p.m.

DAILY: PLAY TIME—Video-game time is the hour before bed.

5. YELLOW LINES AROUND THURSDAY NIGHTS AND SATURDAY AND SUNDAY AFTERNOONS: FAMILY TIME

Do the same with your life, and you can begin watering and fertilizing every plant in the garden of your universe. Commit to this and soon your life will reap a harvest even in places you thought you never had space to grow anything. Also remember: your child will never be more organized than you are! For more information on Time Management and Peace Management, go to www.maximizedliving.com to view the Timesense Guide and *Body by God* book.

LIVIN' IN THE REAL WORLD

At this point you may be wondering, *What does a household with healthy nutritional and lifestyle boundaries look like? How do these lifestyle changes "work" in the real world? And, most important, will it work for my family?*

We talked to one mother who not only manages to raise three healthy kids but heads a successful modeling agency as well. Chantelle Casey, president of American Model & Talent in Granger, Indiana, has a heart for wellness and cultivating inner and outer beauty in others. More than anything else, she says, motivation for positive change has to come from the heart—not a list of rules.

We put some hard questions to Chantelle. The following Q&A shows

---

how this active, real-world mom responded to these tough lifestyle choices and changes.

Q: *How do you create healthy changes in your child's life if he's not naturally inclined in that direction?*

A: This is one of the most critical issues you will ever face as a parent. And if you don't get a grip on it now, [unwholesome tendencies] will get a grip on your children later. Somehow you've got to convey to your children—without blasting their self-esteem—that God loves them no matter what they look like, but that He doesn't want them to go through life unhealthy or unable to play sports with their friends.

The biggest thing for me is that you have to actively participate. My kids get one hour of television per day. A lot of parents view television as a babysitter—GameBoys, TV, DVDs, and electronic gadgets have become addictions for their children. You have to realize that as a parent you're the one who will be responsible to schedule things. Take the time to drive your kids to the beach; in the winter when it's cold, get up off the couch and go out and play with them. That's the Number one thing my husband and I have learned—you've got to set boundaries. In winter, our kids are the only ones outside playing, and the neighbors have commented (wistfully) about it. If playing outside was good enough for us when we were kids, why do we think we can't send our kids outside, even if it's thirty degrees? Buy them warm coats, hats ,and gloves, and send them out! Tell them, "Kids, go make your own fun."

Q: *What if you have a child who is not good at sports and fears ridicule, or it's just not their thing—they would rather stay inside and read or draw pictures. What do you do with a child like that?*

A: I don't force my kids to do anything, but I encourage them to try things, and if they like it they have to make a commitment to stick with it till the end of the season. My oldest son is not an athlete or a bookworm either. He's a musician and plays in a band. To help him get more exercise, we encouraged him to join a baseball team. It took up a big part of our summer driving him to and from games, but we did it because we wanted him to try. He didn't like it, and after the summer we didn't make him go again.

In the meantime we discovered he loves horses, so now we go to a ranch and he rides horses. God wired us all differently, but He definitely didn't wire us to sit on the couch.

Q: *What do you do if your son or daughter is overweight and suffers from very low self-esteem because of it?*
A: One of the things we try to convey to the girls in our modeling agency is that their face is just a gift and to be grateful for that. But who they are on the inside is the real person. Your looks could be gone tomorrow, but the beauty you cultivate on the inside lasts forever. You have to continually tell your children they are wonderful and beautiful and encourage them through the rough times.

Professional counseling may be needed for kids who are truly crippled by low self-esteem, but I believe the best counseling comes from parents. Be there for them.

Q: *How do you create an environment between parent and child so that they feel they can come to you with anything? What types of things open up dialogue?*
A: The two most important things you can do to keep the lines of communication open are (1) *communicate* with your kids, and (2) *respect* your kids—and ask them for mutual respect. Regarding the first point, sit down and have dinner together if you can. Spend time with your children. You can't just let them run hog-wild; kids need to be reined in. Sometimes you may think you're being too hard, too strict, but the kindest thing you can do to your kids is give them boundaries.

On the issue of respect, stop and ask them, "Hey, how was school today?"—and really mean it. So often as parents we just go through the motions. As long as there are no major problems, we let it go. Mutual respect means taking the time to really care and communicate with each other. I'm training my children to communicate with me.

Q: *How do you encourage a child to start looking at life as an adventure— to dream and set goals and have a sense of excitement about what the future holds?*

A: I use everything as an opportunity to tell my kids that God has an awesome plan for their lives. Even if something happens that's bad or slows up our own intentions, it's all part of God's plan. With this mind-set, kids can start to see themselves as truly a work of art—and a work in progress. Their story is not over yet. Sometimes they may feel like the misfit, or the ugly duckling, but remember how that story ends—he grew up to be a beautiful swan.

My family and I were vacationing in Yellowstone Park last summer, and at one point a herd of buffalo was blocking the road. This herd was moving so slowly we were literally stuck there on the road. My husband was frustrated and impatient; I was sort of chilled out. We were on our way to some hot springs later that afternoon, but for now our plans were delayed. When we finally reached the springs, my husband was just in time to save a baby from falling in while his parents weren't looking. If he had not been there at just the right moment, that baby would have drowned. My young son turned to me and said, "Mom, that's why the buffalo were in the road. We needed to be here so Dad could save the baby." There's a lot of peace in knowing that God has us right where we're supposed to be.

Q: *Suppose you're trying to cultivate good nutritional habits in your household but your spouse is not on board. How do you get your husband or wife to participate?*

A: Sometimes you're going to get flack from your spouse, so you want to gradually introduce good food groups. I remember the first time I cooked asparagus and placed it on the table. My husband said, "Ugh. I hate asparagus." I shot him a look. We have a one-bite rule in our household. You have to take one bite, chew it, and swallow it down. You can't spit the food out. If someone really doesn't like a particular food, I don't force it on them, but they have to at least try it. We also don't allow separate meals for our kids.

The good news is that it takes only six to twelve weeks for your taste buds to adapt to a new food—even one you formerly disliked. Sometimes you and your kids may start out eating healthy, then fall back into old habits, like over the holidays when you may eat badly again. The body starts to crave sugars and bad carbs. But within a few days you can get back on track. Realize that the hill is not that steep; it takes only two or three days to get back in a good rut. If I know the goal is attainable, I can get back in the mode where I have a taste for what's healthy and not cookies, cakes, and brownies.

In the same way, a desire for positive change spills over into all areas of life. So don't be surprised if you suddenly see your kids *want* to eat better, exercise more, and get involved with life in a way they never have before.

Take Control of Your Child's Health

Nike was on to something when they coined the slogan "Just Do It." Those three little words are very powerful words. The foundation of this entire book, as you certainly know by now, is that you need to take charge of your child's health and weight problem. The school system isn't going to do it for you; the government isn't going to do it for you. Lasting change is up to you—and your child.

The single most important step you can take to stay in charge of your family's health is to remain informed. Many people read "how-to" information, have great intentions to put it into practice, but then never actually get around to it. Don't let your child be a casualty of "busyness" and the myriad other things that so easily distract us from a worthy goal. And, as we've stated several times in this book, what goal could be more important than the present and future health of your child?

Here's to your success and a lifetime of optimized health for your child!

GET OFF THE BENCH!

I once read a quote that said, "You did not inherit the earth from your parents, it was lent to you by your children." That means the trees, oceans, ozone, and animals were not given to us by our ancestors but lent to us temporarily to give back healthy and intact to our children and grandchildren. The point being, don't destroy the earth!

The same principle applies to our children. They are not ours to ruin. They were lent to us by their children and their children's children. Children are like New Year's resolutions; they're too easy to make and the responsibility necessary to complete the task is rarely carried out. Clearly, we haven't taken this responsibility seriously enough. Our children didn't put themselves here.

If there is something harder than raising children to be exceptional students, to be gentle and caring of their peers, to honor their bodies, to eat well, to exercise, and to be concerned about their future, then I've not seen or heard about it. Young people are always caught up in the dichotomy of trying to be defiant and to fit in at the same time. From the very beginning they are trying to rebel from authority, yet fit in with their friends. All the while they are being influenced by everything from their favorite media idols eating McDonald's and drinking Pepsi to damaging popular trends perpetuated by the "cool" kids or the latest rock, pop, or rap stars.

The job of a parent, teacher, or guardian is tough—really tough—but not impossible. Not impossible at all. Yes, thousands are failing, but thousands are also succeeding in this toughest, but most important, of chores.

Right now your child's taste buds may reject anything not covered in salt, slathered with corn syrup, or preserved with hydrogenated oil. Nonetheless, other than what they do behind your back, they can eat only what you buy or allow on a regular basis. Using the recipes in this book (that you can get from Dr. Mercola, me, or our Maximized Living Mentors), the health-food section of your grocery store, and a little ingenuity, you will find an endless array of snacks, meals, and desserts that kids will enjoy.

Similarly, if kids are used to the various electronic baby-sitters that exist today—computers, TV, video games, cell phones, and whatever else is on its way this Christmas—getting them moving on a regular basis may take nothing less than a chair and a whip. But if electronic hours are planned and not merely allowed, and physical requirements are applied both at home and at school, you can begin to take your child's body away from the technology age. By getting involved with the exercise yourself, you not only create a good model, you get healthier yourself.

The most important hill to take in this battle is our children's minds. With technology doing most of the work, creativity and imagination have run out the door. No wonder learning disorders and depression are at catastrophic levels in our society. Exchanging technology hours for games, crafts, and reading is another critical step in your child's development and their chance for a fulfilling life. It all takes some work, but it's well worth the trade-off. As Winston Churchill said to his troops during World War II, "Do not do what you can, do what you must!" And make no mistake: if you've got kids, the war is on— the war against the dangers of our culture and the fight to give them the future they deserve.

In our Maximized Living Health Centers, we look to help people reach their God-given potential. We combine healthy lifestyle choices, cutting-edge nutritional techniques, spinal corrective care, and a reliance on the body's own natural-healing capabilities into guidelines for raising a fit, healthy child. A healthy, happy child doesn't need to look like Arnold Schwarzenegger or Jennifer Aniston. Attempting to do so typically leads to poor self-image. On the other hand, by exposing your child to the right kind of health care, giving her the opportunity to look her best, and providing her with endless, unconditional love, you do immeasurable good to her confidence and self-esteem. This will speak volumes all throughout her life and allow her to not be average or XL but to in fact *excel.*

Fortunately, the war in America to transform our kids back to health is under way and gaining footholds at the national, statewide, citywide, and school levels. The frightening headlines have at last awakened us, but the pendulum is only slowly swinging the other way.

The list of initiatives required to turn our unhealthy society seems overwhelming. Yet, many around you in your same circumstances and with similar genetics are experiencing health, thinness, and fitness every day. So we know it's completely possible. With awareness and knowledge comes responsibility. Now all it takes is getting off the bench, getting your bat off your shoulder, and swinging away . . . in the right direction.

Although I don't always get it right, I work hard to have three abundantly healthy, fit kids, and in my work I'm surrounded by thousands more. Looking at a world of children who are suffering has given me a burning passion to help. If you're tired and frustrated, and you just don't know where to begin, we're happy to assist you. Look us up at www.maximizedliving.com or www.mercola.com.

Eventually, a society gets the children it deserves.
Let's work together to deserve the best.

The last section of *Generation XL* contains dozens of wholesome, great-tasting recipes. Turn the page to get acquainted with these new, nutritious foods for your family.

KID-PROOF RECIPES

The entire goal of this book has been to introduce you and your child to a new way of living, eating, and moving (exercising) so that together you can find your way into the health and fitness zone and into a lifestyle of optimal health. Since the foods you eat are such a big part of that goal, we've included recipes here that cover the gamut of food choices and taste preferences. And, by the way, the recipes are delicious!

Whole foods were put on this earth for our use. These are not foods that come prepackaged and flash-frozen, are sold over the convenience-store counter, or handed to you through a drive-thru window, but foods that grow in nature. Natural, or whole, foods contain just the right amounts of macronutrients for the proper function of the body, from digestion to elimination.

What's more, whole foods are packed with the enzymes needed to digest the food itself. When you take in food in its natural state, the digestive system will easily break it down, dispense the nutrients to body cells, and quickly eliminate leftover toxins and by-products.

Processed food is anything designed in laboratories, packed for your convenience, zapped with photons, grown in labs, and filled with preservatives so that you can rip it open a year after purchase and nuke it to perfection. Like the flashy packages and containers they come in, processed foods lack life or any truly usable vitamins, minerals, or other nutrients. Anything that is devoid of nutrition or life is unlikely to be able to sustain life.

The farther away you get from eating whole foods, or the farther these foods are from their natural form, the less efficiently the digestive system can break them down—if at all. Processed foods are almost all indigestible. Because these foods cannot pass through the digestive system quickly and cannot be broken down well, they will linger inside your body. This will block the processing of other nutrients, rob you of power, contaminate your organs, create excess fat storage, affect your mood, and contribute to every type of symptom and disease known to humankind.

Not surprisingly, then, this recipe section focuses on eating whole foods and weeding out processed foods. Naturally, you and your child will be tempted to substitute processed foods where it seems most natural. This is understandable if ill advised.

The important thing is to use these recipes. If you do substitute the first time you use a recipe, try following it to the letter the next time. Finally, do a taste comparison. Which version left you and your child feeling fuller, more satisfied, and slightly, if not a whole lot, healthier? Chances are the one made with natural foods will win your vote.

We've thrown a lot at you in this book, but it's important to us that you are not just given the recipes to eat better, but also the tools to eat better for a lifetime. Where the information was available, we've included nutritional analysis and servings information. No matter where you and your child are on the wellness scale, it is important to just start progressing from here, getting 1 percent better each day, enjoying wonderful food, invigorating the body through movement, and experiencing the maximized living you both were intended to live.

Vegetables

Root Vegetables

2	pounds small red potatoes, quartered
1	pound brussels sprouts, halved
½	pound parsnips, peeled and julienned
½	pound carrots, cut into chunks
½	pound turnips, peeled and cut into chunks
⅓	cup olive oil
2	tablespoons horseradish
2	tablespoons vinegar
2	tablespoons snipped fresh dill
½	teaspoon sea salt
¼	teaspoon pepper

Cook vegetables separately in water until tender. Drain. Stir in remaining ingredients.

Combine the vegetables and remaining mixture, toss, and coat.

Zucchini Skilet

⅓	cup chopped onion
3	tablespoons olive oil
3	cups coarsely shredded zucchini
2	teaspoons minced fresh basil
½	teaspoon sea salt
½	teaspoon garlic powder
1	cup diced fresh tomatoes
2	tablespoons sliced, ripe black olives

In a skillet, sauté onion in olive oil. Stir in zucchini, basil, sea salt, and garlic powder.

Cook and stir for 5–6 minutes. Sprinkle with tomatoes and olives. Cover and cook for 5 more minutes.

Squash Medley

3	tablespoons olive oil
1	medium yellow squash, sliced
1	medium zucchini, sliced
¾	pound butternut squash, peeled, seeded, and julienned
1	medium onion, sliced
1	medium green pepper, julienned
1	medium sweet red pepper, julienned
3	garlic cloves, minced
1	tablespoon fresh thyme
¼	teaspoon sea salt
¼	teaspoon pepper

In a skillet, heat the olive oil. Add vegetables, garlic, and thyme. Cook and stir until tender, about 15 minutes. Add sea salt and pepper.

Spinach Bake

1	16-ounce bag frozen chopped spinach
½	cup dairy-free mayonnaise substitute*
1	tablespoon "rice" Parmesan cheese (dairy-free)
½	teaspoon pepper
¼	teaspoon sea salt

*For the best-tasting mayonnaise alternative, we recommend those made with grape-seed oil, such as Vegenaise® brand.

Drain spinach. Mix all ingredients. Microwave on high for 3 minutes. Stir and serve.

Steamed Vegetables

Any vegetables

Lightly steam vegetables. Season with sea salt, pepper, garlic, and onion powder. Sprinkle with "rice" Parmesan cheese (dairy-free).

Grilled Vegetables

2	red peppers, cut in half
2	yellow peppers, cut in half
4	medium zucchini, cut into ½-inch-wide slices
1	cup broccoli florets
1	cup cauliflower

Spray the vegetables with olive oil, season with sea salt and pepper. Grill on both sides 3–4 minutes each.

Asparagus with Red Pepper Sauce

1	teaspoon olive oil
2	large red bell peppers, coarsely chopped, plus thin strips for garnish
2	cloves garlic, minced

1½	pounds asparagus, diced
2	tablespoons red-wine vinegar
1½	tablespoons chopped fresh basil
½	teaspoon sea salt
¼	teaspoon fresh black pepper

In a large skillet heat oil over medium heat. Add the bell peppers and garlic and cook, stirring occasionally, for about 15 minutes. Remove from heat and let cook slightly. In a large saucepan of boiling salted water, cook asparagus for 5 minutes and drain. In a blender purée the bell peppers until smooth. Stir in vinegar, basil, and sea salt. Spoon the red-pepper sauce onto a platter and arrange the asparagus on top. Garnish with bell-pepper strips and chopped basil.

Razzle-Dazzle Skillet

1	cup shredded cabbage
⅓	cup sliced celery
⅓	cup carrots, julienned
2	tablespoons chopped onions
2	tablespoons olive oil
½	teaspoon sea salt
¼	teaspoon pepper
3	tablespoons soy or rice milk
	Minced fresh parsley

Sauté the cabbage, celery, carrots, and onions in olive oil until tender. Sprinkle with salt and pepper. Stir in the milk. Cook for 5 minutes. Sprinkle with parsley.

Hummus Dip and Vegetables

Makes 12 servings. Prep time: 7 min.

1	can garbanzo beans (chick-peas), rinsed and drained
¼	cup tahini butter
3	garlic cloves
2	tablespoons lemon juice
8	sun-dried tomatoes *(optional)* (in oil or reconstituted)

2	tablespoons olive oil
¼	teaspoon salt
¼	teaspoon pepper
1	cup Chinese pea pods
8	mushrooms
2	red bell peppers, sliced
1	cucumber, peeled and sliced
	(Any raw vegetables can be used.)

Combine the first 8 ingredients in a food processor. Use as a dip for the remaining vegetables.

Nutritional Analysis per Serving (4 Tablespoons): Calories: 65, Carbs: 8g, Fat: 4g, Protein: 3g

Quinoa Tabouleh

Makes 4 servings. Prep time: 5 min. Cooking time: 20 min.

½	cup quinoa*
½	teaspoon sea salt
½	teaspoon pepper
⅓	cup tahini butter
	Juice from one lemon
2	cups chopped cucumber
1	cup chopped tomato
1	cup minced parsley

* Quinoa can be found in health-food sections of grocery stores or in health-food markets.

Add quinoa to a saucepan, wash quinoa and drain. Add 1 cup water to quinoa and bring to a boil. Then turn burner to low, cover and simmer for 20 minutes. Cool quinoa. Mix the salt, pepper, tahini, and lemon juice in a food processor until smooth. Combine all ingredients in a bowl and mix well.

Nutritional Analysis per Serving: Calories: 257, Carbs: 23g, Fat: 13g, Protein: 8g

Turkey-Broccoli Statues

Makes 20 servings. Prep time: 5 min. Cooking time: 10 min.
A creative way to get kids to eat their broccoli.

2	pounds fresh broccoli spears
⅓	cup fat-free sour cream
¼	cup Vegenaise (see notes on ingredients)
1	tablespoon thawed frozen orange juice concentrate
1	tablespoon Dijon mustard
½	teaspoon curry
1	teaspoon oregano
1	pound smoked turkey, sliced thinly

Steam broccoli spears until bright green. Cool. Mix the sour cream, Vegenaise, orange juice, mustard, curry, and oregano in a bowl. Slice turkey in 2-inch strips and spread with sour cream. Roll the stalk up in the turkey with the crown part sticking out like a head. Allow the kids to play with the broccoli statues as long as they eat them in the end.

Nutritional Analysis per Serving (2 roll-ups): Calories: 51, Carbs: 4g, Fat: 5g, Protein: 7g

Fermented Vegetables (Kraut)
Makes 30 servings. Prep time: 15 min.

1	head red cabbage
2	heads green cabbage
6	carrots
2	green apples
1	teaspoon salt
	(Can also use celery, kohlrabi, ginger, garlic, seaweeds, pineapple, kale—almost any produce can be fermented.)

It is best to scald all equipment in hot water before using.

Peel 3 outer leaves of each cabbage and set aside. Shred the rest of the cabbage and the above vegetables in a food processor. Take 3 cups of the shredded vegetables and place in a blender with enough water to make a thick juice. Add one teaspoon of salt and blend on HIGH. Add the thick juice to the bowl of shredded veggies and mix well. Add the veggie mixture to 1.5-quart glass jars. Pack them tightly by pushing the material with a wooden spoon. Leave 2 inches of room at the top for the veggies to expand.

Use the cabbage leaves to roll them and put them on top of the jars to keep the jars packed.

Seal the jars with the lids and let sit at room temperature for a week, then put in the fridge. The vegekraut will keep up to one year. The kraut will taste sour. Eat a tablespoon with every meal to aid digestion and bowel and immune system function.

Nutritional Analysis per Serving: Calories: 34, Carbs: 8g, Fat: 0g, Protein: 1.5g

Extraordinary Coleslaw

Makes 4 servings. Prep time: 15 min.

4	cups napa cabbage, shredded
1	red pepper, chopped
½	cup shredded carrot
2	scallions, sliced
¼	cup sliced celery
¼	cup mayonnaise
1	teaspoon tamari (healthy version of soy sauce)
1	teaspoon maple syrup
1	teaspoon grated ginger

Combine the vegetables in a bowl. In a separate bowl, whisk together the mayo, tamari, maple syrup, and ginger. Toss the mayo combination with the coleslaw. If your kids do not like the vegekraut by itself, you can mix some of it in with this coleslaw to temper the sour flavor.

Nutritional Analysis per Serving: Calories: 114, Carbs: 16g, Fat: 7g, Protein: 4g

Cucumber Salad

Makes 8 servings. Prep time: 5 min. Cooking time: 20 min.

3	cucumbers
2	teaspoons diced ginger root
½	cup rice vinegar
1	teaspoon raw honey
1	teaspoon dark sesame oil
2	tablespoons tamari (or soy) sauce

Peel cucumbers and slice very thinly (or use the slicer blade on a food processor). Mix the remaining ingredients well and mix with the cucumbers. Chill for 20 minutes and serve.

Nutritional Analysis per Serving: Calories: 75, Carbs: 9g, Fat: 1g, Protein: 5g

Broccoli Salad

Makes 4 servings. Prep. time: 10 min.

3	cups chopped broccoli
¼	cup chopped red onion
¼	cup crumbled feta or sharp cheddar cheese
6	slices of turkey bacon, cooked and chopped
4	stalks of celery, finely chopped
¼	cup dried cherries, raisins, or cranberries
¼	cup chopped toasted walnuts

Dressing:

¾	cup mayonnaise
1	teaspoon sweetener
1	tablespoon vinegar

Steam broccoli for 1 minute. Place broccoli in the freezer to cool for 1 minute. Mix dressing ingredients. Combine all ingredients with the dressing and toss.

Nutritional Analysis per Serving: Calories: 279, Carbs: 8g, Fat: 25g, Protein: 9g

Asian Asparagus and Seaweed Salad

Makes 4 servings. Prep time: 10 min. Cooking time: 10 min.

Seaweed is such a nutritious food because it is rich in minerals, especially iodine.

1	pound asparagus
½	cup dried seaweed *(optional)* (wakame, arame, kelp)
2	garlic cloves, minced
1	tablespoon grated ginger root
2	tablespoons tamari (or soy) sauce

½	teaspoon sea salt
1	teaspoon honey
¼	teaspoon red pepper flakes
1	teaspoon dark sesame oil
1	tablespoon rice vinegar
⅛	teaspoon cayenne pepper

Soak the seaweed in water for 30 minutes. Add a colander and water to a large pot and bring to a boil. Snap off the ends of the asparagus and slice each stalk into bite-size pieces. Steam until tender (7 minutes). Rinse with cold water. Combine the remaining ingredients in a bowl and toss with the asparagus and seaweed. Can be served hot or cold.

Nutritional Analysis per Serving: Calories: 49, Carbs: 7g, Fat: 2g, Protein: 3g

Summer Vegetables

3	cups cauliflower
2	cups broccoli florets
2	medium carrots, thinly chopped
1	medium zucchini, quartered and thinly chopped
1	medium red onion, julienned
¾	cup vinegar
3	tablespoons honey
½	teaspoon sea salt
2	tablespoons olive oil

In a bowl, combine the first five ingredients, set aside. In a saucepan, heat the vinegar, honey, and salt. Remove from heat, stir in olive oil. Pour over vegetables and toss to coat. Cover and refrigerate overnight. Serve cold.

Marinated Tomatoes

6	large tomatoes
½	cup thinly chopped green onions
½	cup olive oil
¼	cup red-wine vinegar

¼	cup minced fresh parsley
2	garlic cloves, minced
1	teaspoon sea salt
1	teaspoon dried thyme
¼	teaspoon ground pepper

Place tomatoes and onions in a bowl. In a shaker, combine the remaining ingredients.

Shake well. Pour over tomatoes. Cover and refrigerate for one hour.

Broccoli and Cabbage Salad

1	small head of cabbage, shredded
1	bundle of fresh broccoli, chopped
½	cup chopped dates (optional)

Dressing:

1	cup dairy-free mayonnaise substitute*
¼	cup honey
	Juice from one freshly squeezed lemon

*For the best-tasting mayonnaise alternative, we recommend those made with grape-seed oil, such as Vegenaise® brand.

Place cut vegetables in a bowl. Pour the dressing over the vegetables. Mix well.

Tip: Omit the dates for a fantastic alternative to coleslaw. Serve with Sloppy Joes.

Harvest Salad

Dressing:

¼	cup red-wine vinegar
1	teaspoon honey
½	teaspoon sea salt
½	teaspoon dill weed
¼	teaspoon pepper
2	tablespoons olive oil

Salad:

2	cups sliced cucumbers
1	cup sliced red onion, separated into rings
2	medium, ripe tomatoes, cut into wedges
1	cup thinly sliced radish
1	cup cubed avocado

Mix dressing ingredients and pour over combined salad ingredients.

Mixed Green Salad with Egg and Ranch Dressing

Salad:

2	whole boiled eggs and 2 boiled whites cut into slices
2–4	cups of mixed greens
8–10	green olives

Ranch Dressing Dry Mix

1	cup parsley flakes
½	cup minced onions
¼	teaspoon onion powder
¼	cup garlic powder
½	teaspoon sea salt (optional)
¼	teaspoon pepper (optional)
⅛	cup basil
8	ounces dairy-free mayonnaise substitute*

*For the best-tasting mayonnaise alternative, we recommend those made with grape-seed oil, such as Vegenaise® brand.

Mix all dry ingredients for dressing. Put in an airtight container or storage bag to be stored in a cool, dry place. Use this mix any time you need to make a fresh batch of dressing.

Blend 8 ounces dairy-free mayonnaise substitute with 2 tablespoons of ranch dressing dry mix in blender on high. Add water to desired consistency.

Pour over salad and serve.

Caesar Salad

Dressing:

¼	cup red-wine vinegar
1	tablespoon honey
¼	teaspoon sea salt
½	teaspoon pepper
2	tablespoons olive oil
1	tablespoon lemon juice
½	teaspoon minced fresh garlic

Mix dressing ingredients well. Pour over your Caesar salad.

Sassy Salad

3	cups frozen corn, thawed
1½	cups black beans
3	medium tomatoes, diced
1	cup chopped green pepper
1	cup chopped sweet red pepper

Dressing:

¼	cup olive oil
2	tablespoons minced fresh cilantro
1	garlic clove, minced
1	teaspoon sea salt
½	teaspoon pepper
	Juice from one freshly squeezed lemon

Soak black beans overnight in water, rinse and drain. Can substitute one 15-ounce can of black beans.

Combine the first 5 ingredients. Mix dressing and pour over vegetables. Toss and coat. Cover and refrigerate for 1 hour before serving.

Just Like Mashed Potatoes

Makes 4 servings. Prep time: 10 min. Cooking time: 40 min.

Cauliflower belongs to the cruciferous family of vegetables, which are excellent for cancer prevention. (Potatoes, on the other hand, have little nutritional value and are high in carbs.)

1	head of cauliflower cut into small pieces
1	tablespoon butter
¼	cup milk or milk substitute
1	teaspoon Spike seasoning
½	teaspoon pepper

Steam cauliflower in a steamer basket for 40 minutes or until tender. Add cauliflower to the blender with the remaining ingredients and blend. Adjust seasonings if needed. Another topping kids may enjoy on their "mashed potatoes" is lecithin granules, which taste like butter. Lecithin granules are found in health-food stores and are good for optimal brain function.

Nutritional Analysis per Serving: Calories: 60, Carbs: 3g, Fat: 3g, Protein: 2g

Spinach and Cheese

Makes 4 servings. Prep time: 5 min. Cooking time: 10 min.

1	tablespoon butter
1	teaspoon curry powder
¼	cup red onion, minced (Red onion is the healthiest onion due to its color; it's high in flavonoids.)
1	package (10-oz.) frozen spinach, thawed, or 10 oz. fresh spinach, chopped
1	teaspoon salt or Spike
¼	cup low-fat cottage cheese
¼	cup feta cheese (or use another ¼ cup cottage cheese)

Melt butter in a skillet over medium heat. Stir in the curry, onion, spinach, and salt. Cook for 5 minutes. Stir in the cheeses and allow to melt.

Nutritional Analysis per Serving: Calories: 126, Carbs: 4g, Fat: 13g, Protein: 8g

Soup

Quick Beef and Vegetable Soup

Makes 6 servings. Prep time: 10 min. Cook time: 10 min.

1	pound steak, cut into thin strips (or chicken, ostrich, buffalo, etc.)
2	garlic cloves, pressed
2	teaspoons coconut oil, divided
6	cups broth (see "Sauces" section for how to make your own)
16	ounces frozen stir-fry vegetables
2	green onions, sliced thinly
¼	cup stir-fry sauce (comes in a packet with the stir-fry vegetables or choose your own)

In a large pot or Dutch oven, heat the coconut oil on high and tilt the pot to make sure the bottom is evenly covered. Add the garlic and enough beef to create a single layer and allow to cook 1 minute until slightly browned. Then turn the beef over and do the same. Remove from the pot and repeat with the rest of the beef and remaining teaspoon of oil. Set aside.

Add the broth to the pot; cover and bring to a boil over high heat. Add the vegetables; reduce heat to low and simmer for 5 minutes. Add the beef and onions to the pot and heat for another minute.

Nutritional Analysis per Serving: Calories: 160, Carbs: 7g, Fat: 6g, Protein: 19g

Minestrone

Makes 4 servings. Prep time: 5 min. Cooking time: 20 min.

1	cup sliced chicken sausage
1	can garbanzo beans, rinsed and drained
4	cups broth (nonhydrogenated) or water
½	cup tomato puree or pasta sauce
1	small red onion, chopped
2	stalks celery, diced
½	cup diced carrot
½	small zucchini, sliced

3	cloves garlic, pressed
1	cup chopped broccoli
¼	cup dried seaweed *(optional)* (Seaweed increases the nutritional value.)
1	bay leaf
⅓	cup frozen peas
2	tablespoons miso paste*
¼	cup elbow macaroni (preferably a wheat-free kind made from rice or quinoa)
	Salt (to taste)
½	teaspoon pepper

*Miso is a fermented soybean paste, popular in Japan, which aids in digestion and restores the normal flora in the GI tract. All people should eat some kind of fermented foods every day to achieve optimal health.

Fry sausage in a skillet until browned on both sides. Add to a pot, all of the ingredients up until the bay leaf. Simmer for 25 minutes. Add the peas and pasta and cook until the pasta is al dente (10 minutes). Take one cup of the soup broth and blend or whisk it with the miso. Then add it back to the pot. Do not continue to cook the soup after the miso has been added as boiling temperatures kill the healthy bacteria in the miso. Add salt (if needed) and pepper to taste.

Nutritional Analysis per Serving: Calories: 227, Carbs: 28g, Fat: 4g, Protein: 18g

World's Easiest Chili

Makes 8 servings. Prep time: 5 min. Cooking time: 10 min.

1	pound lean ground beef, ostrich, or bison
1	24-ounce jar of mild, medium, or hot chunky salsa (to taste)
2	15-ounce cans black beans
2	8-ounce cans tomato sauce
1	tablespoon chili powder
	Add sautéed: mushrooms, carrots, celery, or diced broccoli or cauliflower to increase the nutritional value of the chili *(optional)*.

Cook beef on medium-high heat until browned. Drain excess fat from the meat. Drain 1 can of beans and mash. Add all ingredients to a big pot and mix together. Heat on medium until heated through. Do not serve with crackers. It is important to start to wean carbohydrate-addicted kids off their high-grain, high-sugar diets. In addition, wheat is the highest allergenic food.

Nutritional Analysis per Serving: Calories: 267, Carbs: 22g, Fat: 12g, Protein: 14g

Thai Coconut Soup

Makes 4 servings. Prep time: 10 min. Cooking time: 20 min.

1	tablespoon butter
2	garlic cloves, pressed
½	cup red onion, chopped
2	teaspoons ground lemon grass
⅛	teaspoon cayenne pepper
½	cup chopped mushrooms
1	tablespoon grated ginger root
1	tablespoon fresh lime juice
1	whole chicken, cooked
1	can coconut milk
2	cups chicken stock (recipe below) or use organic chicken stock from a health-food store
1	teaspoon honey or sugar
¼	cup chopped cilantro
2	tablespoons fish sauce

Remove the meat from the bone and cut into small pieces. To make chicken stock, place chicken bones and skin in 3 cups water with 2 teaspoons salt and boil for 20–30 minutes, or until the stock is reduced to 2 cups. In a medium saucepan, melt butter on medium heat. Add garlic, onion, lemon grass, and cayenne, and sauté for 1 minute. Add mushrooms and ginger and sauté for 1 minute. Add lime juice and sauté for 1 minute. Add chicken and coconut milk and bring to a slow boil. Then add stock, honey, cilantro, and fish sauce. Simmer for 10 minutes.

Nutritional Analysis per Serving: Calories: 265, Carbs: 6g, Fat: 19g, Protein: 13g

Italian Spinach Soup

Meatball Mixture:

1	egg
½	cup rice Parmesan cheese (dairy-free)
1	small onion, chopped
1	teaspoon pepper
1	teaspoon garlic powder
2	pounds ground turkey

Soup Mixture:

2	quarts vegetable broth*
1	cup chopped spinach
1	teaspoon onion powder
1	tablespoon chopped parsley
1	teaspoon sea salt
½	teaspoon pepper
½	teaspoon garlic powder

*Vegetable broth can be made from scratch by boiling onion, celery, carrots, garlic clove, sea salt, and pepper. (Add other vegetables as desired.) A quicker alternative is to purchase organic vegetable bouillon cubes or organic vegetable broth in the carton—available at your local health-food store.

Meatballs

In a bowl, thoroughly mix all ingredients for meatballs. Shape into 1-inch balls. In microwave, cook them on high for 3–4 minutes, drain.

Soup

In a large pot, add all ingredients for the soup mixture. Add the meatballs and bring to a boil. Simmer uncovered for 10 minutes and serve.

Garden Soup

1	pound ground turkey
1	cup chopped onion

4	medium tomatoes, chopped
2	cups frozen corn
2	cups water
3	tablespoons chopped fresh parsley
3	tablespoons Italian seasoning
1	teaspoon sea salt
½	teaspoon pepper

Cook turkey, onion, and garlic over medium heat. Drain. Add remaining ingredients. Bring to a boil. Simmer uncovered for 30 minutes.

Chicken Soup with Broccoli, Spinach, and Cauliflower

6	cups chicken broth
1	skinless, boneless whole-chicken breast
1	yellow onion, finely diced
½	cup broccoli florets
½	cup cauliflower florets
½	cup chopped spinach
3	tablespoons finely chopped fresh parsley

Add sea salt and fresh ground pepper to taste. In a large saucepan bring chicken broth to a simmer. Add the chicken breast and simmer just until tender and no trace of pink remains, 8–10 minutes. Remove the chicken breast. Transfer to a cutting board and cut into 1-inch cubes. Set aside. Add the onions, broccoli, cauliflower, and chopped spinach to the broth. Simmer for 10 minutes. Add the cubed chicken, parsley, sea salt, and pepper. Simmer 3 more minutes.

Breakfast Dishes

Carob Muffins

1	cup oat flour
¾	cup whole wheat flour (finely sifted)
¼	cup carob powder
1	tablespoon baking powder

2	egg whites or 1 egg
¼	cup honey
3	tablespoons olive oil
1	cup soy, rice, or almond milk
1½	teaspoons pure vanilla extract
⅔	cup carob chips

Preheat oven to 400°. Line muffin tin with muffin cups. In a bowl, mix all dry ingredients. In a blender, mix all wet ingredients. Add this mixture to the dry ingredients. Fold in the carob chips. Divide mixture evenly into prepared muffin cups. Bake 15 minutes (or until toothpick inserted into the middle of a muffin comes out clean). Remove muffins and place on a rack to cool.

Applesauce Muffins

1	cup whole wheat flour (finely sifted)
½	cup oat bran
1½	teaspoons baking soda
1	teaspoon ground cinnamon
¼	teaspoon ground cloves
½	teaspoon ground nutmeg
¼	teaspoon ground allspice
¼	cup soy, rice, or almond milk
2	egg whites or 1 egg
1	cup applesauce (unsweetened)
2	tablespoons olive oil
2	teaspoons pure vanilla extract
¼	cup molasses
¼	cup raisins

Preheat oven to 375°. Line 8 muffin cups with muffin papers. In a bowl, mix all dry ingredients, excluding raisins. In a blender, mix all wet ingredients. Add this mixture to the dry ingredients. Fold in the raisins. Divide mixture evenly into prepared muffin cups. Bake 20–25 minutes. Remove muffins and place on rack to cool.

Blueberry Muffins

1	cup whole wheat flour (finely sifted)
½	cup oat bran
2	teaspoons baking powder
¼	cup honey
2	egg whites or 1 egg
2	tablespoons olive oil
½	cup apple juice
2	teaspoons pure vanilla extract
1	teaspoon lemon juice
1	cup fresh or frozen blueberries

Preheat oven to 375°. Line 8 muffin cups with muffin papers. In a bowl, mix all dry ingredients, excluding the blueberries. In a blender, blend all wet ingredients. Add to the dry ingredients. Fold in the blueberries. Divide mixture evenly into prepared muffin cups. Bake for 20 minutes. Remove muffins and place on rack to cool.

Crock-Pot Oatmeal

1½	cups rolled oats
3½	cups water
1	large apple, unpeeled, chopped
¼	cup raisins
3	tablespoons honey (optional)
1½	teaspoons ground cinnamon
1	teaspoon pure vanilla extract

In a Crock-Pot, combine all ingredients. Turn on low setting. Cover and cook overnight (6–8 hours).

Baked Oatmeal

1½	cups oatmeal
½	cup honey

½   cup soy, rice, or almond milk

¼   cup olive oil

1   teaspoon baking powder

¼   teaspoon sea salt

1   teaspoon pure vanilla extract

       warm or cold soy, rice, or almond milk *(optional)*

       fresh fruit for topping *(optional)*

Combine first seven ingredients. Mix well. Spread evenly in a 13 x 9 x 2-inch baking pan. Bake at 350° for 30–35 minutes. Immediately spoon into bowls. Add milk or fruit if desired.

Apple Oatmeal

2½   cups water

2   large, sweet apples, unpeeled, coarsely shredded

1⅓   cups rolled oats

¼   teaspoon ground cinnamon

¼   teaspoon ground nutmeg

In a saucepan, combine water and apples. Bring to a boil.

In a small bowl, combine oats and spices. Mix well. Stir into boiling water. Reduce heat to medium-low and cook 5 minutes, stirring frequently. Serve hot. Sprinkle lightly with maple syrup.

Orange Oatmeal

½   cup water

1   cup orange juice (unsweetened)

⅔   cup rolled oats

Bring water and orange juice to a boil in a saucepan. Stir in oats. Cook 5 minutes, stirring frequently. Remove from heat, cover, let stand 5 minutes. Serve hot.

Overnight Oatmeal

1½	cups rolled oats
¼	cup golden raisins
1	large apple (chopped)
3¾	cups water
1½	teaspoons cinnamon
⅛	teaspoon nutmeg
2	tablespoons ground or crushed flaxseeds
1	teaspoon pure vanilla extract
3	tablespoons honey *(optional)*
2	teaspoons chopped almonds, hazelnuts, or walnuts *(optional)*

In a large Crock-Pot, combine all ingredients. Turn on low setting. Cover and cook overnight (6–8 hours).

Pancakes

Makes 6–8 pancakes.

½	cup oat flour*
½	cup whole wheat flour (sifted)
2	teaspoons baking powder
1	tablespoon honey
1	cup soy, rice, or almond milk
1	tablespoon lemon juice
1	tablespoon olive oil
2	egg whites or 1 egg
1	teaspoon pure vanilla extract

*Oat flour: Pour oatmeal into blender and blend on high until you have oat flour.

In a bowl, mix all dry ingredients. In a blender, blend all wet ingredients, and then add to the dry ingredients. Mix well. Preheat a nonstick pan, lightly oiled. Drop batter onto pan, using 2 tablespoons for each pancake. Turn pancakes when bubbles form on the top side. Cook until golden brown on both sides. Serve hot.

Overnight Waffles

4	cups oatmeal*
¼	cup whole wheat flour
1	tablespoon plus 1 teaspoon baking powder
2	teaspoons ground cinnamon
4	cups soy, rice, or almond milk
3	tablespoons olive oil
2	teaspoons pure vanilla extract

*Oatmeal = rolled oats

Mix all dry ingredients in a bowl. Blend all wet ingredients in a blender, and then add to dry ingredients. Cover and chill overnight. To prepare: Preheat a well-oiled waffle iron. Batter should be thick. Spoon batter onto hot iron. Close iron and cook 4–6 minutes. Drizzle lightly with pure maple syrup or top with your favorite fruit topping. (Waffles can be refrigerated or frozen and later reheated or toasted.)

Homemade Strawberry Jam

1	cup honey
2	tablespoons fresh lemon juice
1	cup water
16	ounces strawberries, fresh or frozen (cut into small pieces)
5	teaspoons plain gelatin (flavorless)*

* Available in health-food stores, made from plants

Put all ingredients in a saucepan. Let mixture come to a boil, then simmer on medium heat for 1 hour, stirring frequently. Pour into jars and refrigerate.

Homemade Bread

5/8	cup soy or rice milk
¾	cup water
1½	tablespoons olive oil

3	tablespoons honey
4	cups whole wheat flour (finely sifted)
1½	teaspoons sea salt
2½	teaspoons instant yeast
¼	cup sunflower seeds *(optional)*

You will need a bread machine for this recipe.

Put wet ingredients into bread-machine pan. Add the dry ingredients, adding yeast last. Set on "rapid," "white bread," or "wheat bread" setting.

Oat Biscuits

1¾	cups whole wheat flour (finely sifted)
¼	cup oat bran
1	tablespoon plus 1 teaspoon baking powder
¼	teaspoon sea salt
4	tablespoons olive oil
¾	cup soy or rice milk

Preheat oven to 450°. Lightly oil baking sheet. In a bowl, mix all dry ingredients. Add oil mix with a fork or pastry blender, until mixture resembles coarse crumbs. Add milk. Stir until moistened. Place dough on floured surface and knead a few times, until dough holds together in a ball. Place a sheet of waxed paper over dough and roll to ¼-inch thick. Remove waxed paper and fold dough in half (now ½-inch thick). Using a 3-inch biscuit cutter (or a glass) cut dough into 10 biscuits. Place on prepared baking sheet. Bake 10 minutes or until bottoms of biscuits are lightly browned. Remove from oven and let cool. Serve warm.

Granola

2¼	cups oatmeal
¼	cup wheat germ
¼	cup oat bran
¼	cup honey
1½	teaspoons ground cinnamon
½	cup orange juice

2	tablespoons olive oil
1	teaspoon pure vanilla extract
1½	teaspoons almond extract
	Add carob, walnuts, raisins, sunflower seeds, or any dry food to the mix *(optional)*.

Preheat oven to 300°. Lightly oil a 10 x 15-inch pan. Mix all dry ingredients in a bowl. Blend all wet ingredients in a blender, and then add to the dry ingredients. Mix well. Spread mixture evenly in prepared pan. Bake 30–35 minutes or until light brown, stirring every 10 minutes. Be careful not to burn. Remove from oven and break up any lumps. Cool in pan. Store in container.

Vegetable Omelet

1	tablespoon olive oil
1	cup sliced fresh mushrooms
1	cup sliced zucchini
4	eggs, slightly beaten
¼	teaspoon black pepper
3	tablespoons water
½	tablespoon olive oil
½	cup rice mozzarella shredded (optional)

In a skillet heat olive oil, add mushrooms and zucchini. Cook over medium heat until vegetables are crisply tender (4–5 minutes). Remove from skillet and set aside. In a small bowl stir together remaining omelet ingredients except olive oil and cheese. In same skillet heat olive oil. Pour egg mixture into skillet. Cook over medium heat, lifting with a spatula to allow uncooked portion to flow underneath until omelet is set (3–4 minutes). Place sautéed vegetables and cheese on half of omelet. Gently fold other half of omelet over filling.

Tip: For even fluffier omelets, add ⅓ cup water or soymilk to the egg mixture before cooking. Beat thoroughly.

Spinach & Mushroom Omelet

½	cup fresh mushrooms
¼	cup chopped onion

1	cup fresh spinach leaves
1	tablespoon olive oil
3–4	eggs, slightly beaten
⅛	teaspoon sea salt
⅛	teaspoon pepper

In a skillet sauté the mushrooms, onions, and spinach leaves until tender, remove from skillet. In a small bowl stir together the remaining omelet ingredients except olive oil. In the same skillet, heat olive oil. Pour egg mixture into skillet. Cook over medium heat, lifting slightly with spatula to allow uncooked portion to flow underneath, until omelet is set (3–4 minutes). Place sautéed mushrooms and spinach on half of omelet. Gently fold other half of omelet over filling. Serve hot.

Tip: For even fluffier omelets, add ⅓ cup water or soymilk to the egg mixture before cooking. Beat thoroughly.

Apple Oat Pudding

1	cup rolled oats
½	teaspoon baking soda
1	teaspoon ground cinnamon
½	teaspoon ground nutmeg
1	large sweet apple, unpeeled, shredded (1 cup)
3	egg whites
⅓	cup molasses
⅔	cup water
1	tablespoon lemon juice

Preheat oven to 325°. Lightly oil a 1-quart baking pan. In a large bowl, combine oats, baking soda, cinnamon, and nutmeg. Mix well. Add apple, mix. In a small bowl combine the remaining ingredients, whisk until blended. Add to oat mixture, mix well. Place mixture into prepared pan. Cover lightly with foil. Place in a larger pan and pour enough water in the large pan to come halfway up the side of the pan with pudding. Bake 1 hour. Serve warm.

Fruit Oat Pudding

1½	cups rolled oats
1¼	cups orange juice
½	cup applesauce
¼	cup raisins
1	teaspoon ground cinnamon
1	teaspoon pure vanilla extract
½	teaspoon almond extract
¼	cup fruit-only raspberry jam

Preheat oven to 350°. Lightly oil 1-quart baking pan. In a large bowl, combine all ingredients. Mix well. Place into prepared pan. Bake uncovered for 40 minutes. Serve hot or cold.

Overnight Muesli

4	tablespoons rolled oats
1	tablespoon golden raisins
6	tablespoons milk (almond, rice, soy, or oat milk)
1	small apple
2	teaspoons chopped almonds or hazelnuts
1	teaspoon honey
¼–½	cup honey (optional)

Put oats and raisins in a bowl, add the milk, then cover and leave in refrigerator overnight. Next day, grate the apple and stir in the nuts and honey.

Oat Bran Breakfast Treat

1½	cups water
½	cup oat bran
1	tablespoon cornstarch
¼	cup water
2	tablespoons honey

1½	teaspoons pure vanilla extract
¼	teaspoon almond extract
¼	teaspoon ground cinnamon
¼	cup raisins
¼	cup slivered almonds
	Raspberry jam to taste

Line a 4 x 8-inch loaf pan with plastic wrap, letting the edges hang over the sides of the pan. Bring the 1½ cups of water to a boil. Add oat bran, stirring briskly with a fork or wire whisk. Cook 3 minutes or until thick, stirring frequently. Remove from heat.

In another small saucepan combine cornstarch and ¼ cup water, stirring until cornstarch is dissolved. Add honey, extracts, and cinnamon. Cook over medium heat, stirring until it comes to a boil. Boil, stirring for 1 minute. Add cornstarch mixture, raisins, and almonds to oat bran. Mix well. Spoon mixture into prepared pan. Let cool, then cover and leave overnight. To serve, invert mold onto a serving plate, remove plastic wrap, and cut into 4 servings. Top with raspberry jam.

Lunch Dishes

Broccoli & Spinach Omelet

2	tablespoons olive oil
1	cup fresh spinach leaves
1	cup fresh small broccoli florets, cut into small pieces
3	eggs, slightly beaten
¼	teaspoon sea salt
¼	teaspoon pepper
3	tablespoons water
1	teaspoon olive oil
½	cup shredded rice mozzarella cheese (optional)

In a skillet heat the olive oil. Add spinach leaves and broccoli. Cook until crisply tender (4–5 minutes). Remove from skillet and set aside. In a small bowl stir together remaining omelet ingredients except olive oil and cheese.

In same skillet heat 1 teaspoon olive oil. Pour egg mixture into skillet. Cook over medium heat, lifting slightly with a spatula to allow uncooked portion to flow underneath, until omelet is set (3–4 minutes). Place sautéed vegetables and cheese on half of omelet. Gently fold other half of omelet over filling. Serve hot.

Tip: For even fluffier omelets, add ⅓ cup water or soymilk to the egg mixture before cooking. Beat thoroughly.

Spinach & Tomato Omelet

1	teaspoon olive oil
1	cup fresh spinach leaves
3 or 4	eggs, slightly beaten
⅛	teaspoon sea salt (optional)
⅛	teaspoon pepper (optional)
1	large tomato, chopped

In a skillet beat the spinach leaves until tender. Remove from skillet and set aside. In a small bowl stir together the remaining omelet ingredients except olive oil and tomatoes. In the same skillet heat 1 teaspoon olive oil. Pour egg mixture into skillet. Cook over medium heat, lifting slightly with a spatula to allow uncooked portion to flow underneath, until omelet is set (3–4 minutes). Place sautéed spinach leaves and chopped tomatoes on half of omelet. Gently fold other half of omelet over filling. Serve hot.

Tip: For even fluffier omelets, add ⅓ cup water or soymilk to the egg mixture before cooking. Beat thoroughly.

Veggie Pan Pizza

Dough:

1	cup whole wheat flour (finely sifted)
½	cup oat bran
1	teaspoon baking powder
½	teaspoon sea salt
¾	cup plus 1 tablespoon water

Sauce:

½ cup crushed tomatoes
¼ teaspoon Italian seasoning

Topping:

⅔ cup shredded rice mozzarella cheese
3   tablespoons each finely chopped onion, mushrooms, and green pepper

Preheat oven to 400°. Lightly oil a 10-inch heavy cast-iron skillet.

To prepare crust: in a large bowl combine dry ingredients and mix well. Add water and stir. Place dough in prepared skillet. Press in pan. Bake 10 minutes. Remove pan from oven.

To assemble pizza: Combine tomato sauce and spices. Spread evenly over dough, staying ½ inch away from edge of pan. Sprinkle cheese and the vegetables evenly over sauce.

Bake 15 minutes. Remove from skillet.

Potato Wedges

3½ tablespoons "rice" Parmesan cheese (dairy-free)
1 tablespoon dried basil
1 tablespoon freshly minced parsley
¼ teaspoon salt
¼ teaspoon pepper
1 very large baking potato, cut into wedges (not peeled)
2 teaspoons olive oil in a bowl

Combine "rice" Parmesan cheese, basil, salt, and pepper. Brush cut sides of potato wedges with olive oil, then dip into cheese mixture. Bake uncovered at 400° for 25 minutes.

Calypso Rice

3 cups water
1 medium onion
2 celery sticks, thinly chopped

2	medium carrots, thinly chopped
1	cup each frozen corn, peas, and cut green beans
1	tablespoon olive oil
1	teaspoon sea salt
½	teaspoon chopped garlic
¼	teaspoon pepper
1½	cups brown rice, uncooked

In a saucepan, combine the water, vegetables, and olive oil. Bring to a boil. Add rice. Reduce heat, cover, and let simmer for 20 minutes.

Rice with Beans

1¾	cups shredded rice mozzarella cheese
6	ounces cooked brown or wild rice
1½	cups sliced fresh mushrooms
½	cup chopped onion
½	cup chopped green pepper
½	cup chopped sweet red pepper
1	tablespoon olive oil
15	ounces (1½ cups) black beans, cooked and drained
½	cup frozen corn
½	cup frozen peas
2	teaspoons Italian seasoning
	Sea salt and pepper to taste

Cook the rice according to package directions. Meanwhile, in a skillet sauté mushrooms, onions, and peppers in olive oil until crisp-tender. Add the beans, 1 cup shredded cheese, corn, peas, Italian seasoning, salt, and pepper. Stir in rice. Transfer to a 3-quart baking dish. Sprinkle with remaining cheese. Bake uncovered at 350° for 30–35 minutes.

Wild Rice

1	cup wild rice, cooked
2	tomatoes, diced
¾	cup small broccoli florets

1⅓	cups green lentils
½	cup shredded rice mozzarella
1	bay leaf
2	tablespoons olive oil
2	tablespoons lemon juice
1	minced garlic
2	tablespoons chopped mint
1	tablespoon chopped parsley
½	teaspoon sea salt
¼	teaspoon pepper

Put lentils in a saucepan with the bay leaf and cover generously with water. Bring to boil and simmer 25 minutes. Drain well. Steam broccoli until tender, drain. Whisk together the oil, lemon juice, garlic, salt, and pepper. Pour over hot lentils and mix well. Stir in mint, parsley, broccoli, tomatoes, and mozzarella and mix well. Serve over cooked wild rice.

Tip: Lentils can be soaked overnight to save time.

Mexican Rice

1	cup brown rice, cooked
1	package Mexican rice seasoning*
2	tomatoes, diced
½	cup sliced black olives

*Organic mixes without unnecessary chemicals and preservatives, such as Bearitos® brand, can be found in your local health-food store.

Cook rice. Add seasoning mix. Mix well. Fold in tomatoes and black olives.

Oven-Baked Potatoes

12	medium potatoes, peeled and cubed
¼	cup rice Parmesan cheese (dairy-free)
2	teaspoons sea salt
1	teaspoon garlic powder
1	teaspoon paprika
½	teaspoon pepper
¼	cup olive oil

Place potatoes in ziplock bag. Combine the remaining ingredients. Add to potatoes and shake to coat.

Pour potatoes onto baking pan. Bake uncovered at 375° for 40–50 minutes.

Spinach Lasagna

1	pound firm tofu
4–5	ounces cooked lasagna noodles (whole wheat)
5	ounces fresh spinach leaves
8	slices rice mozzarella cheese (dairy-free)
4	large tomatoes (cubed and crushed in blender)
1	tablespoon Italian seasoning
1	teaspoon sea salt
1	teaspoon pepper
1	teaspoon honey

Preheat oven to 375°. Drain all moisture from tofu. Crumble into mixing bowl, seasoning with a dash of sea salt and pepper and set aside. Mix crushed tomatoes with Italian seasoning, sea salt, pepper, and honey. Place 1 cup of tomato sauce in the bottom of the baking dish. Add a layer of noodles, followed by ½ cup of tofu crumbles. Add 1 cup of spinach leaves over tofu. Add a layer of mozzarella slices. Repeat layers, starting with sauce again, until the pan is full. Press layers down. Press any remaining sauce over the top. Cover with foil and bake for 35 minutes.

Splendid Spaghetti

1	box whole wheat spaghetti
6	large tomatoes, crushed in a blender
3	tablespoons Italian seasoning
1½	teaspoons sea salt
¼	teaspoon pepper
1	tablespoon honey
½	pound soy browned ground beef substitute*

*Can be found at your local grocer or health-food store. We recommend Yves® Veggie Cuisine brand Ground Round.

Cook spaghetti and drain.

Mix crushed tomatoes with seasonings in a bowl. Brown veggie ground round in a saucepan. Add tomato sauce. Heat thoroughly. Serve over spaghetti.

Veggie Sandwiches

1	loaf whole wheat bread, sliced
	Tomatoes, sliced to taste
	Cucumbers, sliced to taste
	Dairy-free mayonnaise substitute* to taste
	Sea salt to taste
	Pepper to taste

*For the best-tasting mayonnaise alternative, we recommend those made with grape-seed oil, such as Vegenaise® brand.

Spread mayonnaise substitute onto slices of bread. Top with tomato and cucumber slices.

Sprinkle with sea salt and pepper to your liking.

Zucchini Boats

2	medium zucchini
¾	pound ground turkey
1	small onion, chopped
½	cup sliced fresh mushrooms
½	cup chopped sweet red peppers
½	cup chopped green peppers
1	cup shredded rice cheese
2	tablespoons ketchup
½	teaspoon sea salt
¼	teaspoon pepper

Trim the ends of the zucchini. Cut in half lengthwise. Scoop out pulp, leaving a ½-inch shell. Finely chop pulp. In a skillet, cook ground turkey, zucchini pulp, onion, mushrooms, and peppers until meat is brown, drain. Remove from heat. Add ½ cup "rice" cheese, ketchup, sea salt, and pepper. Mix well. Spoon into the zucchini shells. Place in a greased 13 x 9 x 2-inch baking pan. Sprinkle with remaining cheese. Bake uncovered at 350° for 30 minutes.

Tuna Salad in a Pita

⅓	cup dairy-free mayonnaise substitute*
½	teaspoon garlic salt
½	teaspoon lemon pepper
6	ounces white tuna
¼	cup chopped celery
1	hard-boiled egg, chopped
2	tablespoons finely chopped green onion
2	tablespoons finely chopped green pepper
1	cup shredded lettuce
2	tablespoons finely chopped cucumber

*For the best-tasting mayonnaise alternative, we recommend those made with grape-seed oil, such as Vegenaise® brand.

Roasted Eggplant Sandwich

3	pounds eggplant (about 2 large peeled and cut into 1/2-inch slices)
	Sea salt to taste
3	medium shallots, finely chopped
1	medium garlic clove, minced
¼	cup red-wine vinegar
⅛	cup extra-virgin olive oil
¼	teaspoon pepper
½	tablespoon fresh basil, finely chopped
2	red sweet peppers, cut into halves

Preheat oven to 400°. Place the eggplant pieces in a large colander and sprinkle with sea salt evenly. In a large roasting pan, stir together the shallots, garlic, vinegar, olive oil, and pepper. Place the eggplant slices and peppers into the roasting pan and coat evenly. Place in the oven and roast for about 30 minutes, turning once. Serve on a grain roll, topped with feta cheese.

Turkey Burger with Grilled Zucchini and Red Pepper

1	pound ground turkey
1	large zucchini, sliced

2	red peppers, cut into strips
2	green onions, chopped
½	tablespoon olive oil

Season ground turkey with sea salt and pepper, then form into patties. Grill or pan-fry until done. In olive oil, sauté zucchini, red peppers, and green onions. Top each turkey patty with sautéed vegetables. Serve with a salad.

Garden Tuna Melt

¼	cup chopped celery
¼	cup dairy-free mayonnaise substitute*
6	ounces drained tuna
4	sprouted grain rolls, split and toasted
8	green pepper rings
8	slices ripe tomato
8	slices rice cheese (mozzarella)
2	tablespoons chopped green onions

*For the best-tasting mayonnaise alternative, we recommend those made with grape-seed oil, such as Vegenaise® brand.

Heat oven to 350°. In a medium bowl stir together celery, mayonnaise substitute, and tuna. Place rolls on cookie sheet. Spread tuna mixture on rolls. Layer each with one green pepper ring and one tomato slice. Bake for 10–12 minutes. Remove from oven. Top with one slice of rice cheese. Garnish with green onion. Continue baking for 1–2 minutes or until cheese melts.

Turkey Breast / Vegetable Stir-Fry

1	tablespoon cornstarch
1	tablespoon honey
¾	teaspoon green ginger
½	teaspoon chili powder
¼	teaspoon garlic powder
¼	teaspoon pepper
½	cup cold water
¼	cup soy sauce
1	pound turkey breast, cut into three strips

2	tablespoons olive oil
2	cups cauliflower
1	large onion, chopped
1	cup sliced carrots

In a small bowl, whisk together the first eight ingredients until smooth, then set aside. In a skillet, stir-fry turkey in olive oil for 3–5 minutes. Add broccoli, cauliflower, onion, and carrots to soy sauce mixture. Cover and cook for 8 minutes, stirring occasionally.

Wild Rice Grilled Vegetables

2	medium zucchini
2	medium eggplants
6	plum tomatoes
2	medium carrots
2	yellow sweet peppers

Trim the stems off the zucchini and eggplants and carrots. Cut them lengthwise into ¼-inch-thick slices. Cut plum tomatoes in half, cut peppers in half and spray with olive oil. Grill for 5 minutes on each side. Serve over wild rice.

Main Dishes

Teriyaki Salmon

¼	cup olive oil
¼	cup fresh lemon juice
¼	cup soy sauce
1	teaspoon mustard
1	teaspoon ground ginger
¼	teaspoon garlic powder
4	salmon steaks

In a ziplock bag, combine the first 6 ingredients. Mix well. Set aside ¼ cup for basting and refrigerate. Place the salmon into the ziplock bag and let marinate for 1 hour in the refrigerator. Drain and discard marinade. Place the salmon on a broiler pan or grill. Broil or grill for 4–5 minutes. Brush with reserved marinade. Turn and broil or grill for 5 more minutes or as desired.

Tip: Add a slice of grilled pineapple.

Grilled Salmon with Zucchini

2	pounds salmon or 4 salmon steaks
1	tablespoon olive oil
2	teaspoons lemon pepper
2	red peppers, cut in half
2	yellow peppers, cut in half
4	medium zucchini, cut into ½-inch-wide slices
1	cup broccoli florets
1	cup cauliflower

Marinate salmon in 1 tablespoon olive oil. Baste the salmon on both sides. Grill, turning once, 10 minutes on each side. Spray the vegetables with olive oil, season with sea salt and pepper. Grill on both sides 3–4 minutes each.

Grilled Salmon & Asparagus with Red Pepper

1	tablespoon olive oil
2	chopped shallots
¼	cup fresh lemon juice
4	teaspoons honey
¼	teaspoon cayenne pepper
1	tablespoon chopped fresh ginger
¼	cup red-wine vinegar
2	tablespoons soy sauce
2	tablespoons chopped fresh cilantro
2	pounds salmon or 4 salmon steaks

Sauce: Mix first 8 ingredients in a saucepan until shallots are soft (about 3 minutes). Remove from heat. Mix in cilantro. Baste the salmon on both sides. Grill 10 minutes on each side, turning once and basting frequently with sauce.

Grouper with Mixed Green Salad

1	grouper fillet (large)
1	teaspoon freshly chopped parsley
1	teaspoon freshly chopped dill
1	teaspoon freshly chopped basil
1	teaspoon freshly chopped chives
2	teaspoons dairy-free mayonnaise substitute*

Salad:

2	cups mixed greens
1	cut-up avocado
½	cup cut-up asparagus tips
⅛	cup sesame seeds

*For the best-tasting mayonnaise alternative, we recommend those made with grape-seed oil, such as Vegenaise® brand.

Grilled Salmon

1½	pounds fresh salmon

Coating:

½	teaspoon lemon-pepper seasoning
½	teaspoon sea salt
¼	teaspoon garlic powder

Seasoning:

¼	cup honey
3	tablespoons vegetable broth
3	tablespoons soy sauce
3	tablespoons finely chopped green onion

Option: Place salmon in broiler at 350° for 20 minutes.

Mix coating ingredients in ziplock bag. Coat salmon.

Mix seasoning ingredients in ziplock bag. Shake to mix.

Pour seasoning mixture over salmon or place salmon directly in bag and toss to coat. Refrigerate for 1 hour. Drain and discard marinade. Place salmon skin down on grill over medium heat. Cover and cook for 20 minutes.

Flounder Bake

4	flounder steaks
1	cup dairy-free mayonnaise substitute*
1	tablespoon freshly chopped parsley
1	tablespoon thinly sliced green onion
1	tablespoon chopped fresh dill
½	teaspoon sea salt
¼	teaspoon pepper

*For the best-tasting mayonnaise alternative, we recommend those made with grape-seed oil, such as Vegenaise® brand.

Mix ingredients. Spread mixture over flounder and bake at 350° for 20 minutes.

Herbed Turkey Breast

¼	cup olive oil
⅛	cup lemon juice
2	tablespoons soy sauce
2	tablespoons finely chopped green onion
1	tablespoon rubbed sage
2	teaspoons Italian seasoning
¼	teaspoon pepper
1	whole turkey breast with bones (5–6 pounds)

In a small saucepan, combine the first 7 ingredients. Bring to a boil. Remove from heat. Place turkey in a roasting pan and baste with herb mixture. Bake uncovered at 325° for 1–2 hours, basting every 30 minutes.

Option: Use a rotisserie in place of oven.

Zucchini Chicken Dinner

¾	pound chicken breast, cubed or cut into strips
2	tablespoons olive oil
1	large onion, chopped
2	garlic cloves, minced
2	large tomatoes, puréed in blender

½   teaspoon crushed dried rosemary
½   teaspoon dried oregano
½   teaspoon sea salt
¼   teaspoon cayenne pepper (optional)
3   medium zucchini, halved and cut into ¼ to ½-inch slices

In a skillet over medium heat, cook chicken in olive oil until brown. Add onions and garlic. Add puréed tomatoes and seasoning. Simmer uncovered for 5 minutes. Add zucchini. Cook and stir until crisp-tender.

Chicken Fajita-Style

¾   cup lemon juice
½   cup olive oil
3   garlic cloves, minced
2   teaspoons dried oregano
1   teaspoon ground cumin
½   teaspoon pepper
1½ pounds boneless, skinless chicken breast, cut into thin strips
3   small zucchini, julienned
2   small yellow summer squash, julienned
2   medium green peppers, julienned
2   medium sweet red peppers, julienned

Combine the first 6 ingredients. Divide the mixture between two large ziplock bags. Add chicken to one and vegetables to the other and turn. Refrigerate for 2 hours. Drain chicken and vegetables, discarding marinade. In a skillet, sauté chicken for 5 minutes.

Remove chicken and keep warm. Sauté vegetables in skillet for 3 minutes and drain. Spoon chicken into the skillet with the vegetables. Serve.

Vegetable/Turkey Stir-Fry on Rice Pasta

1   pound ground turkey
1   large onion
4   garlic cloves, minced
¾   cup bean sprouts
4   ounces sliced mushrooms
1   cup corn, fresh or frozen

1   cup broccoli florets
¼   cup soy sauce
2   teaspoons ground ginger

In a large skillet, cook turkey, onion, and garlic over medium heat until cooked through, then drain. Add bean sprouts, mushrooms, corn, and broccoli. Cook for 3–5 minutes. Stir in the soy sauce and ginger. Serve over rice pasta* and toss to coat.

*Pasta made from rice flour found in your local health-food store.

Chicken Stir-Fry over Rice Pasta

2   cups chicken broth
¼   cup cornstarch
3   tablespoons soy sauce
½   teaspoon ground ginger
1   pound boneless, skinless chicken breast, cut into ½-inch strips
2   garlic cloves, minced
½   cup thinly sliced onions
½   cup thinly sliced carrots
3   cups broccoli florets
1   cup fresh or frozen snow peas

In skillet, heat 3 tablespoons of broth. Meanwhile, combine the cornstarch, soy sauce, ginger, and remaining broth until smooth and set aside. Add chicken to the skillet. Stir-fry over medium heat until no longer pink. Remove with a slotted spoon and keep warm. Add garlic, carrots, and onion to skillet. Stir-fry for 3 minutes. Add broccoli and peas. Stir-fry for 5 minutes. Stir broth mixture. Add to skillet with the chicken. Cook and stir for 2 minutes. Serve over rice noodles.*

57   *Noodles made from rice flour found in your local health-food store.

BBQ Chicken with Vegetables

2   pounds cut-up white meat chicken breast
1   tablespoon olive oil

½   cup chopped onion

½   cup chopped green pepper

½   cup thinly sliced celery

½   cup ketchup

¼   cup water

1½   tablespoons honey

1½   tablespoons Worcestershire sauce

¼   teaspoon sea salt

⅛   teaspoon pepper

8   ounces frozen corn

In a skillet, brown chicken in olive oil, transfer to an ungreased 13 x 9 x 2-inch baking dish. Sauté in the skillet onions, green peppers, and celery until tender. In a bowl combine the ketchup, water, honey, Worcestershire sauce, salt, and pepper. Add sauce to vegetables. Bring to a boil. Pour over chicken. Cover and bake 18–20 minutes at 350°. Sprinkle with corn. Bake 20 minutes longer. Serve with salad.

Turkey Roll

1½   pounds ground turkey

1   teaspoon sea salt

¼   teaspoon pepper

Filling:

1½   cups frozen corn

1   egg

¼   cup minced fresh parsley

½   teaspoon sea salt

⅛   teaspoon pepper

Mix turkey with sea salt and pepper. Mix filling ingredients in a separate bowl. Place turkey mixture on a piece of heavy-duty foil and press with hands into a 12 x 10-inch rectangle. Spoon the filling over the turkey mixture, within one inch of the edge. Roll up (jellyroll-style), starting with the short side and peeling foil away while rolling. Seal seams and ends. Place on greased 13 x 9 x 2-inch baking pan. Bake uncovered at 350° for 1 hour.

Mini Meat Loaf

2	pounds ground turkey
1½	teaspoons sea salt
1	teaspoon pepper
1	teaspoon paprika
1	tablespoon freshly chopped parsley
1	onion, chopped
1	egg (optional)

Mix all ingredients well. Roll into 10 equal balls, flattened a little. Fry in pan, turning once.

Turkey Skillet

1	pound ground turkey
1	large onion, chopped
1	large green pepper, chopped
½	large red pepper, chopped
1	teaspoon sea salt
1½	teaspoons chili powder
1	teaspoon dried basil leaves
2	garlic cloves, minced
1½	cups soaked kidney or black beans
½	cup drained reserve liquid (or 8-ounce can organic kidney or black beans)
1½	cups corn (frozen)
⅓	cup sliced black olives
¼	cup chopped parsley

Brown meat in a large skillet. Break into small pieces. Add onions, green peppers, and red peppers. Cook until vegetables are tender-crisp. Gently stir in sea salt, chili powder, basil, garlic, beans, and corn. Simmer for 5–10 minutes. Stir in some or all of the reserved bean liquid if you want to increase moistness. Gently stir in the olives and parsley. Heat through and serve.

Pizza Crust Dough

1	cup whole wheat flour (finely sifted)
½	cup oat bran
1	teaspoon baking powder
½	teaspoon sea salt
¾	cup plus 1 tablespoon water

Preheat oven to 400°. Lightly oil a 10-inch heavy cast-iron skillet. In a bowl, combine dry ingredients. Mix well. Add water. Stir until all ingredients are moistened. Place dough in prepared skillet. Press in pan, wetting hands slightly to avoid sticking. Bake 10 minutes. Remove pan from oven. Top with your favorite toppings. Bake for another 15 minutes. Serve right from the skillet.

Ground Turkey with Vegetables

2	pounds ground white-meat turkey breast
3	medium zucchini, julienned
4	medium carrots, julienned
1	medium onion, cut into three wedges
¾	cup green peppers, julienned
1	garlic clove, minced
1	medium tomato, cut into wedges
½	cup snap peas
½	cup broccoli
1	teaspoon sea salt
1	teaspoon ground cumin

In a skillet, cook turkey over medium heat until no longer pink. Drain. Add the zucchini, carrots, snap peas, onions, green peppers, broccoli, and garlic. Cook and stir for 3–4 minutes or until crisp-tender. Add the tomato, salt, and cumin. Cook 2 minutes longer.

Sloppy Joes

1	pound ground turkey
½	cup chopped celery
⅓	cup chopped green pepper
⅓	cup chopped onion
4	medium tomatoes, crushed in blender
½	tablespoon sea salt
⅛	tablespoon pepper

Sauce:

½	cup ketchup
3	teaspoons honey
1	teaspoon mustard
1½	tablespoons vinegar
1	tablespoon Worcestershire sauce
¼	teaspoon garlic powder

Side Dish: Cole Slaw

1	small head cabbage
1	small bundle broccoli
¼	cup honey
	Juice from 1 freshly squeezed lemon
1	cup dairy-free mayonnaise substitute*

*For the best-tasting mayonnaise alternative, we recommend those made with grape-seed oil, such as Vegenaise® brand.

Brown onion and turkey and drain. In a saucepan, cook green peppers for 2 minutes in a little water, then drain and add to turkey. Add the rest of the ingredients to the turkey mixture. Cook for 1 hour and stir often.

Mix sauce ingredients and add to the boiling Sloppy Joe mixture. Cook another ½ hour.

Shred the cabbage and chop the broccoli. Add Vegenaise® and mix well.

Vegetarian Spaghetti Sauce

1	medium sweet red pepper, chopped
1	medium onion, chopped

4	garlic cloves, minced
2	tablespoons olive oil
1	tablespoon chili powder
1	teaspoon ground cumin
1	teaspoon dried oregano
2	cups cubed, peeled butternut squash
4	large tomatoes cut up into small pieces

In a large saucepan, sauté red pepper, onion, and garlic in oil until tender. Stir in chili powder, cumin, oregano, butternut squash, and tomatoes and bring to a boil. Reduce heat, cover, and simmer for 10–15 minutes or until squash is tender. Serve over rice spaghetti.* Serve with fresh green salad.

*Spaghetti made from rice flour can be found in your local health-food store

Creamy Crispy Chicken Salad

4	fully cooked chicken breasts, shredded
½–1	cup chopped celery
½	cup chopped or sliced almonds
½	cup dairy-free mayonnaise substitute*

*For the best-tasting mayonnaise alternative, we recommend those made with grape-seed oil, such as Vegenaise® brand.

In a large mixing bowl, combine all ingredients. Hand-mix thoroughly with a strong fork. Serve on whole wheat bread slices or pitas.

Tip: In a hurry? Look for canned chicken breast in water at your local health-food store or grocer.

Chicken Salad

Makes 6 servings. Prep time: 10 min.
(The perfect use for leftover meat)

2½	cups cooked chicken (turkey, roast beef, hard-boiled eggs, fish, etc.)
½	cup mayonnaise (we recommend Vegenaise made with grape-seed oil or make your own)
1	tablespoon lemon juice
2	tablespoons curry powder

⅛	cup diced red onion
½	cup diced celery
¼	cup chopped almonds
1	tablespoon capers
	Dash of cayenne pepper
	Lettuce or bitter greens for serving

Mix all the ingredients together and chill 1 hour before serving. Serve on a bed of romaine lettuce or mixed greens. (Red leaf, bitter tastes: kale, radicchio, arugula, dandelion. It is a good idea to include bitter tastes in your child's diet. Even if s/he doesn't like the taste at first, you can mix it in with other greens to temper the bitterness. Bitter foods are excellent for improving digestion and cleansing the liver and are missing in most American diets.)

Nutritional Analysis per Serving: Calories: 208, Carbs: 3g, Fat: 20g, Protein: 11g

Mexican Salad

Makes 4 servings. Prep time: 10 min.

1	head romaine lettuce, torn into pieces
4	chicken breasts (or ostrich, steak), grilled and chopped
1	tomato, chopped
⅓	cup chopped red onion
2	ounces black olives, sliced
¼	cup natural ranch salad dressing
¼	cup salsa
4	tablespoons guacamole
½	cup chopped cilantro

In a large bowl, toss all the ingredients above the dividing line. Serve the guacamole and cilantro in separate bowls on the side.

Nutritional Analysis per Serving: Calories: 240, Carbs: 8g, Fat: 12g, Protein: 27g

Chinese Salad

Makes 4 servings. Prep time: 10 min.

| 1 | cup mung bean sprouts |
| 2 | cups chopped cooked chicken or ostrich |

5	ribs bok choy, chopped
5	ribs napa cabbage, chopped
2	scallions, minced
½	cup shredded carrots
¼	cup roasted peanuts
¼	cup chopped cilantro
⅔	cup Chinese Dressing (see Sauces section, page 225)

Mix all the ingredients together and spoon the dressing on the salad. Salad will keep for 2 days without dressing.

Nutritional Analysis per Serving: Calories: 275, Carbs: 6g, Fat: 17g, Protein: 23g

Tuna Salad

4	cups shredded lettuce
4	plum tomatoes, sliced
½	cucumber, sliced
2½	ounces sliced olives
12	ounces solid white tuna, chunked
1	tablespoon minced fresh parsley

Arrange lettuce on plate. Top with tomatoes, cucumbers, olives, and tuna. Drizzle Lemon Dressing (see page 222) over salad. Sprinkle with parsley.

Vegetable Chicken Salad

Salad

2	cups cauliflower
4	cups torn fresh spinach
1	cup broccoli florets
1	cup sliced cucumbers
2	cups mixed green salad
1	large chicken breast cut into cubes

Dressing

| ⅓ | cup olive oil |
| ⅓ | cup lemon juice |

½   teaspoon sea salt
¼   teaspoon nutmeg
½   teaspoon minced fresh garlic

Mix salad with dressing and add cut-up chicken breast.

Mahimahi Mixed Green Salad
Marinade

2   garlic cloves, minced
1   chopped shallot
6   tablespoons fresh lemon juice
¼   cup olive oil
½   teaspoon sea salt
¼   teaspoon pepper

Salad

4   cups shredded lettuce
4   plum tomatoes, sliced
½   cucumber, sliced

Mix marinade ingredients well. Pour over mahimahi. Cover and refrigerate for 2 hours. Grill for 5–6 minutes on each side. Add mahimahi to salad ingredients, serve with Lemon Dressing (see page 222).

Meat and Vegetable Kabobs
Makes 4 servings. Prep time: 10 min. Cooking time: 15 min.

1   pound chicken breast (ostrich, steak, salmon) cut into 1½–inch pieces
½   cup pineapple chunks
2   small zucchini, cut into 1-inch chunks
1   cup red and yellow bell pepper chunks
8   mushrooms
8   cherry tomatoes
2   tablespoons wheat-free tamari or soy sauce
2   tablespoons dry sherry or white wine
1   teaspoon dark sesame oil

3   garlic cloves, pressed

2   scallions, cut into 1-inch pieces

5   wooden skewers

Add all ingredients to a plastic bag. Marinate 1–4 hours in the refrigerator. Soak 5 (12-inch) skewers in water for 25 minutes. Thread the chicken and vegetables on the skewers. Place skewers on the rack of a broiler pan 5 inches from the broiler. Brush with marinade. Broil for 5 minutes. Turn kabobs over and brush with marinade and broil for 5 more minutes.

Nutritional Analysis per Serving: Calories: 142, Carbs: 8g, Fat: 3g, Protein: 18g

Stir-Fry

Makes 4 servings. Prep time: 15 min. Cooking time: 10 min.

2   tablespoons coconut oil

1   pound chopped meat of your choice: chicken, ostrich, beef, fish, tempeh (soy product)

2   garlic cloves, pressed

1   cup sliced red onion

2   peppers, cut into strips

4   stalks of celery, chopped

1   cup chopped broccoli

½   cup broth

2   tablespoons teriyaki sauce (MSG-free)

1   teaspoon soy sauce

2   tablespoons cornstarch, arrowroot, or kudzu (for thickening)

In a large skillet, wok, or pot, heat 1 tablespoon oil and add the meat and garlic. Cook the meat until browned. Remove the meat and set aside. Add the vegetables to the skillet. Cover and steam for 5 minutes. Add the browned meat back to the skillet with the broth, teriyaki sauce, and salt, and continue cooking uncovered for 5 minutes. Mix the cornstarch with ¼ cup cold water and stir into the skillet until it thickens. Serve over brown rice or cauliflower rice.

Nutritional Analysis per Serving: Calories: 300, Carbs: 11g, Fat: 15g, Protein: 30g

Cauliflower Rice

Makes 4 servings. Prep time: 5 min. Cooking time: 5 min.

Cauliflower rice looks and tastes like white rice but is nutrient-dense and will not cause blood sugar increases, sleepiness, or constipation as white rice does. Another way to use this is to combine it half and half with cooked brown rice, which will decrease the carb count by half.

1	head cauliflower

Finely chop cauliflower in the food processor. Steam or sauté in butter for a few minutes until tender. Add any of the following to season: butter, soy sauce, Spike, lecithin granules (taste like butter).

Nutritional Analysis per Serving: Calories: 30, Carbs: 5g, Fat: 0g, Protein: 0g

Thai Curry

Makes 4 servings. Prep time: 10 min. Cooking time: 20 min.

2	tablespoons coconut oil
2	tablespoons green or red curry paste
2	cups sliced chicken breast
2	tablespoons fish sauce
1	14-ounce can coconut milk
1½	cups stir-fry vegetables of your choice
1	cup sweet peas
2	green chilies, cut lengthwise

Heat the oil in a wok. Stir-fry green curry paste for 1 minute. Add chicken and fish sauce. Stir-fry until chicken is cooked. Add coconut milk and bring to boil. Add vegetables, sweet peas, and green chilies. Cook for 3–5 minutes. Remove from heat. Serve with cauliflower rice. Coconut milk, green curry paste, green chilies, and fish sauce may be purchased at an Oriental market.

Nutritional Analysis per Serving: Calories: 375, Carbs: 8g, Fat: 28g, Protein: 24g

Spaghetti Squash with a Red Meat Sauce

Makes 2 servings. Prep time: 10 min. Cooking time: 35 min.

Spaghetti squash is a yellow oblong squash that when cooked and scraped out with a fork, resembles strands of spaghetti. It is much lower in carbs than pasta and much higher in nutrition. We recommend using Beano™ with this product as it may cause gas.

1	spaghetti squash
1	cup Newman's Own spaghetti sauce (low in sugar)
½	pound ground beef (or ground ostrich or turkey)
	Salt, pepper to taste

*If your kids do not like spaghetti squash, you can also try making your own "pasta" using zucchini and the Spiral Slicer.™

Preheat oven to 375°. Cut the spaghetti squash down the middle and scoop out the seeds. Place facedown on a greased baking tray and bake for 35 minutes. Cool for 5 minutes and scrape the insides with a fork to remove the long strands. Brown the ground beef, season with salt and pepper, drain excess fat. Heat the pasta sauce in a saucepan over medium heat. Add the cooked ground beef. Pour over the squash.

Nutritional Analysis per Serving (2 servings): Calories: 190, Carbs: 8g, Fat: 23g, Protein: 20g

Mediterranean Shrimp

Makes 6 servings. Prep time: 20 min. Cooking time: 25 min.
This recipe is fast and easy!

2	tablespoons olive oil
2	cloves garlic, pressed
1	medium red onion, chopped
1	cup finely chopped broccoli
1	small can of mushrooms, sliced
4	medium tomatoes, diced
1½	pounds frozen, cooked, shelled, de-veined shrimp, thawed or cooked scallops
1	teaspoon salt or Spike
½	teaspoon pepper
	Dash of cayenne pepper
½	teaspoon rosemary
5	tablespoons balsamic vinegar
½	cup crumbled feta cheese

Preheat oven to 350°. Heat the oil in a large skillet on medium. Sauté the onions and garlic until translucent; add the broccoli, mushrooms, and tomatoes and simmer on medium-low heat for 10 minutes. Add the remaining ingredients up to the feta cheese and heat through for 5 minutes. Pour into a greased casserole dish and sprinkle with feta cheese. Bake for 5 minutes.

Nutritional Analysis per Serving: Calories: 200, Carbs: 7g, Fat: 7g, Protein: 27g

Poached Eggs and Spinach

Makes 2 servings. Prep time: 15 min. Cooking time: 15 min.

This is a tasty, easy one-dish supper. Eggs are best eaten raw, boiled, or poached, as cooking at high temperatures (for scrambled eggs or omelets) harms the delicate proteins in the eggs.

1	tablespoon butter or coconut oil
½	cup red onion, minced
1½	cups chopped broccoli
6	mushrooms, sliced
½	teaspoon sea salt or herbamare
½	teaspoon black pepper
	Dashes of cayenne or ¼ cup salsa
½	teaspoon oregano
½	teaspoon basil
½	medium tomato, chopped
½	cup diced zucchini, yellow squash, or bell pepper
1	cup chopped spinach
¼	cup sour cream
4	large eggs

In a large skillet, sauté the onion in the butter over medium heat for 4 minutes. Add the broccoli, mushrooms, and salt. Cook and stir for 5 more minutes. Add the herbs, zucchini, and tomato. Cook for 5 minutes. Stir in spinach and sour cream. Increase the heat to medium-high. With a large spoon, indent the veggies to make 4 beds for each egg. Break an egg in each bed. Cover and poach for 5 minutes or until just set.

Nutritional Analysis per Serving: Calories: 334, Carbs: 15g, Fat: 23g, Protein: 17g

Turkey Casserole

Makes 6 servings. Prep time: 20 min. Cooking time: 25 min.
This is a great recipe for using leftover baked turkey or chicken.

2	cups cooked small pieces of turkey
½	cup diced carrots
2	cups diced celery
¼	cup minced whole scallions
½	apple, chopped
½	cup mayonnaise
1	tablespoon lemon juice
¼	cup chopped canned pimiento
½	cup chopped almonds
¼	cup cheese of your choice

Preheat the oven to 350°. Combine the first 7 ingredients in one bowl and spread in a greased 2-quart casserole dish. Sprinkle the almonds and cheese on top. Bake 25 minutes or until heated through.

Nutritional Facts per Serving: Calories: 276, Carbs: 6g, Fat: 20g, Protein: 18g

Sauces

Vinaigrette

1	shallot, chopped
1	medium garlic clove, minced
1	tablespoon chopped fresh parsley
1	tablespoon chopped fresh basil
1	teaspoon mustard
1	tablespoon fresh lemon juice
3	tablespoons red-wine vinegar
¾	cup olive oil
½	teaspoon sea salt
¼	teaspoon pepper

Mix in blender.

Creamy Veggie Dip

1	cup dairy-free mayonnaise substitute*
2	teaspoons fresh horseradish

*For the best-tasting mayonnaise alternative, we recommend those made with grape-seed oil, such as Vegenaise® brand.

Vigorously mix ingredients. Keep refrigerated. Enjoy!

Hummus Spread

1	1-pound can chickpeas (garbanzo beans), rinsed or drained (or soak dry beans)
1	tablespoon lemon juice
¼	teaspoon sea salt
2	cloves garlic, minced

In a blender, combine all ingredients and blend until smooth. Spoon into a bowl. Cover and chill. Serve cold on sandwiches, crackers, or whole wheat pita bread.

Lemon Dressing

¼	cup red-wine vinegar
1	tablespoon honey
¼	teaspoon sea salt
½	teaspoon pepper
2	tablespoons olive oil
1	tablespoon lemon juice
½	teaspoon minced fresh garlic

Mix well.

Hot Strawberry Syrup

1	16-ounce package frozen or 1 pint fresh strawberries
2–3	tablespoons honey

If using frozen strawberries, make sure they are thoroughly thawed. Heat strawberries and honey in saucepan until hot. Do not boil. Pour into blender. Mix for 1 minute on lowest setting. Serve immediately.

Shitake Gravy

Makes 4 servings. Prep time: 10 min. Cooking time: 10 min.

This is a wonderful recipe because it is delicious, wheat-free, and contains shitake mushrooms, which are great for the immune system.

¼	cup minced red onion
½	teaspoon pressed garlic
⅓	cup shitake mushrooms, minced (fresh or dried and reconstituted—cheaper)
2	tablespoons coconut oil or butter
2½	tablespoons wheat-free flour (wheat-free baking mix, amaranth, rice, potato)
2	cups broth or water
1	teaspoon sea salt, herbamare, Spike

Sauté the onion, garlic, and mushrooms in ½ tablespoon oil until the onions are translucent and transfer to a bowl. Melt the remaining oil and quickly stir in the flour. Very slowly add broth, stirring constantly. Add salt or seasoning to taste.

Nutritional Analysis per Serving: Calories: 104, Carbs: 2g, Fat: 15g, Protein: 4g

Spinach Dip

Makes 4 servings. Prep time: 15 min.

Can be served warm or cold. Great for dipping raw vegetables or as a topping for cooked vegetables.

8	ounces frozen spinach, chopped, steamed, and drained (retain ¼ cup liquid)
1	tablespoon chopped chives, scallions, or red onion
¼	cup minced celery
2	tablespoons butter
¼	cup grated Parmesan cheese
¼	cup sour cream or yogurt
1	garlic clove, pressed
1	teaspoon wheat-free tamari (alternative to soy sauce)
	Pepper to taste

Drain spinach into a colander and squeeze to remove water (collect the water in a bowl underneath). In a medium saucepan, sauté chives in butter until soft. Turn heat to low and add remaining ingredients, stirring until creamy.

Nutritional Analysis per Serving: Calories: 122, Carbs: 3g, Fat: 11g, Protein: 4g

Guacamole

Makes 4 servings. Prep time: 8 min.

1   ripe avocado (soft when pressed)
½   tablespoon fresh lemon juice
2   tablespoons salsa
¼   teaspoon garlic salt
1   tablespoon fresh cilantro
1   garlic clove

Scoop out avocado into a food processor. Add remaining ingredients and blend well. Leftover guacamole can be stored in a small bowl, with the avocado pit in the middle and plastic wrap pressed on top of the surface of the guacamole to prevent browning.

Nutritional Analysis per Serving: Calories: 50, Carbs: 3.5g, Fat: 4g, Protein: 1g

Berry Salsa

Makes 4 servings. Prep time: 10 min.
Serve with grilled chicken, pork, or fish.

1   cup chopped strawberries
⅓   cup chopped blueberries
¼   cup chopped red bell pepper
1   tablespoon chopped red onion
¼   cup chopped carrot
2   teaspoons cider vinegar
1   teaspoon honey
1   teaspoon minced jalapeno pepper
⅛   teaspoon ground ginger

Combine all ingredients in a bowl and allow flavors to blend for 20 minutes before serving.

Nutritional Analysis per Serving: Calories: 22, Carbs: 6g, Fat: <1g, Protein: <1g

Chinese Dressing
Makes 4 servings. Prep time: 10 min.

4	tablespoons olive oil
2	tablespoons sesame oil
¼	cup rice vinegar
1	tablespoon fresh lime juice
1	teaspoon red pepper flakes
1½	tablespoons wheat-free tamari (or soy sauce)
1	tablespoon minced ginger root
1	garlic clove, pressed
1	teaspoon honey
1	tablespoon sesame seeds
	Salt and pepper to taste

Mix ingredients. Makes about 1 cup. Olive oil will turn cloudy when refrigerated so allow to warm to room temperature before serving or run the bottle under hot water to warm.

Nutritional Analysis per Serving: Calories: 250, Carbs: 3g, Fat: 27g, Protein: 0g

Broths

Prep time: 15 min. Cooking time: 30–120 min.

It is preferable to make your own broth because most commercial broths are pasteurized; contain preservatives, MSG, and hydrogenated oils; and are more expensive than making your own. After straining the broth, refrigerate it overnight and skim off the layer of fat on the surface (meat broths only). Freeze the broth in ice-cube trays and store in a ziplock bag. Six cubes equal 1 cup of broth. The vegetables from the vegetable broth recipe can be added to the chicken and beef recipes for added flavor and nutrition.

Chicken broth: Place chicken bones and skin from 1 chicken in 7 cups of water, add 3½ teaspoons salt. Boil until the water is reduced to 6 cups (30 minutes).

Beef broth: Take 4 pounds of meaty beef bones and roast them in a pan at 450° F for 25 minutes until brown. Transfer to a large pot. Add 3 quarts water, bring to a boil, and turn down to a simmer and cover for 2 hours.

Vegetable broth: Boil in 1 gallon water any of the following ingredients about 45–60 minutes: greens that surround the cauliflower and cabbage, tops of celery, onions, shriveled-up carrots and other veggies that got lost in the refrigerator, onion, garlic, parsley, salt, and pepper, plus any herbs you happen to like, tomatoes, seeded and coarsely chopped; celery stalks, thickly sliced; carrots, peeled or thickly sliced; leeks, white part only; turnips, pepper, zucchini, garlic, 2 sprigs Italian parsley, 1½ teaspoons dried thyme, 2 bay leaves, 10 black peppercorns.

Snacks and Treats

Peanut Raisin Clusters

½	cup oatmeal
½	cup coarsely chopped peanuts (unsalted)
½	cup raisins or dates
½	cup chopped, mixed dried fruit
½	teaspoon pure vanilla

Combine all ingredients in a food processor. When mixture holds together, roll into 24 one-inch balls. Cover and chill.

Candy Balls

½	cup oatmeal
3	tablespoons peanut butter, smooth or crunchy*
1	teaspoon pure vanilla
¼	teaspoon almond extract
2	tablespoons orange juice
1	teaspoon honey
2	tablespoons soy, rice, or almond milk

*You can substitute almond or soy butter for peanut butter.

In a bowl, mix all ingredients. Mix well. Divide mixture evenly and roll into 12 balls.

Cover and store in refrigerator.

Piecrust

⅔   cup oatmeal flour
½   cup whole wheat flour (finely sifted)
½   teaspoon baking powder
¼   cup plus 1 tablespoon soy or rice milk (ice cold)
3   tablespoons olive oil

Mix all dry ingredients in a bowl. With a fork, stir in milk and oil. Work dough into a ball. Rolling dough between two sheets of waxed paper, form a 12-inch circle. Carefully remove top sheet of waxed paper and insert crust into pie pan. Fit crust in pan, leaving a little overhang. Carefully remove remaining waxed paper. Bend edges of crust under and flute dough with fingers or a fork. For no-bake filling, prick bottom and sides of crust about 40 times with a fork. Bake crust in oven for 10 minutes at 450°. Cool before filling.

Soft Pretzels

11   cups water
3   cups whole wheat flour (finely sifted)
2   tablespoons olive oil
1   tablespoon honey
2   teaspoons instant yeast
1   teaspoon sea salt
2½   tablespoons baking soda
    Coarse salt, to taste (optional)

You will need a bread machine for this recipe.

Put all wet ingredients in bread machine pan. Add dry ingredients to the pan, adding yeast last. Select "dough" setting.

When dough is done, remove from bread pan and place on an oiled countertop. Gently roll and stretch dough into 12-inch ropes. With a sharp knife, divide dough into 4 or 5 equal pieces. Roll each piece into 14-inch ropes. Shape into a pretzel. Set aside pretzels on oiled countertop, cover with a towel, and let rise, until doubled in size or about 20 minutes.

Meanwhile, in a large pot, bring water and baking soda to a boil. Reduce heat to a gentle simmer. Preheat oven to 425°. Gently lift pretzels on a slotted spoon into water for 20 seconds. Turn over and repeat for 20 seconds. Remove from water and place on rack, allowing dough to drain. After all are done being soaked, bake on a cookie sheet for 15–20 minutes or until golden brown. Serve warm.

Banana Bread

¾   cup oat bran
1¼   cups whole wheat flour (finely sifted)
1   teaspoon baking soda
1   teaspoon baking powder
¼   cup chopped walnuts (optional)
½   cup honey
2   tablespoons olive oil
2   egg whites or 1 egg
¼   cup soy, rice, or almond milk
1½   teaspoons pure vanilla extract
2   medium bananas (very ripe)

Preheat oven to 350°. Lightly oil tube pan or bread pan. Mix all dry ingredients, excluding bananas, in a bowl. Blend all wet ingredients and bananas in a blender. Add to the dry ingredients and mix well. Spoon mixture into prepared pan. Bake 30 minutes. Place pan on rack to cool.

Cranberry Crisp

2   cups cranberries, fresh or frozen
2   medium apples, unpeeled, chopped (2 cups)
¼   cup honey

Topping:

¾   cup rolled oats
2   tablespoons whole wheat flour (finely sifted)
1   teaspoon cinnamon
2   tablespoons honey
1   tablespoon olive oil
1½   tablespoons apple juice

Preheat oven to 350°. Lightly oil a 9-inch pie pan. In a saucepan combine the cranberries, apples, and honey. Cool over medium heat, stirring frequently for 5–10 minutes, until cranberries pop. Remove from heat, spoon into prepared pan.

To prepare topping:

In a bowl combine oats, finely sifted flour, cinnamon, and honey. Mix well. Add oil and apple juice and mix well. Distribute evenly over cranberry mixture. Bake uncovered 30 minutes or until lightly brown. Serve warm or cold.

Granola Bars

1½	cups rolled oats (oatmeal)
¼	cup oat bran
¼	cup finely chopped almonds
½	teaspoon ground cinnamon
2	tablespoons plus 1 teaspoon olive oil
⅓	cup honey
½	teaspoon pure vanilla extract
¾	teaspoon almond extract

Preheat oven to 350°. Lightly oil a baking sheet. Mix all dry ingredients in a bowl. Add oil, honey, vanilla, and almond extract. Mix until all ingredients are moistened. Place mixture on prepared sheet and press into the shape of a rectangle. Wet hands lightly while working mixture. Bake 12 minutes. Remove from oven and cut into 16 bars with a very sharp knife. Separate bars slightly and return to oven for 5 more minutes. Remove from oven and place on wire rack to cool.

Strawberry Jam Bars

¾	cup whole wheat flour (finely sifted)
1	cup rolled oats
¼	cup oat bran
½	teaspoon baking powder
¼	cup honey
2	tablespoons olive oil
½	cup apple juice
1	teaspoon pure vanilla extract
⅓	cup fruit-only strawberry jam

Preheat oven to 350°. Lightly oil an 8-inch square pan. In a large bowl combine finely sifted flour, oats, oat bran, and baking powder. Mix well.

In another bowl combine honey, oil, apple juice, and vanilla. Add to dry mixture and mix well. Set aside ½ cup of oat mixture.

Press remaining mixture firmly in the bottom of prepared pan. Spread jam evenly over oat mixture. Drop remaining mixture evenly over jam. Press down lightly into the jam. Bake 20 minutes. Cool in pan. Cut into squares.

Apple Bars

¾	cup whole wheat flour (finely sifted)
¼	cup oat bran
1	teaspoon baking powder
1	teaspoon ground cinnamon
3	tablespoons chopped walnuts
¼	cup honey
½	cup apple juice
1½	teaspoons pure vanilla extract
1	tablespoon olive oil
1	large apple, unpeeled, chopped

Topping:

1½	teaspoons honey
¼	teaspoon ground cinnamon

Preheat oven to 350°. Lightly oil 8-inch square baking pan. In a bowl combine finely sifted flour, oat bran, baking powder, cinnamon, walnuts, and honey. Mix well. In another bowl combine remaining ingredients except apple. Add to dry mixture along with apple. Mix well.

Spread dough into prepared pan. Bake for 35 minutes. Cool in pan. Spread topping over cooled cake. Cut into bars.

Carrot Bars

1	cup whole wheat flour (finely sifted)
½	cup oat bran
1	teaspoon baking soda

1	teaspoon baking powder
2	teaspoons ground cinnamon
⅛	teaspoon ground allspice
¼	cup raisins (optional)
3	tablespoons chopped walnuts
1	cup crushed pineapple
2	egg whites
1½	teaspoons pure vanilla extract
½	cup honey
2	cups finely shredded carrots

Preheat oven to 350°. Lightly oil an 8-inch square pan. In a large bowl combine finely sifted flour, oat bran, baking soda, baking powder, and spices. Mix well. Add raisins and walnuts.

In a blender, combine remaining ingredients except carrots. Blend. Add to dry ingredients along with carrots. Mix well.

Spoon into prepared pan. Smooth the top. Bake 50 minutes. Cool in pan. Cut into bars.

Berry Almond Oat Bars

2–2½	cups rolled oats
¼	cup oat bran
1	teaspoon baking powder
¼	cup honey
1	cup apple juice
2	tablespoons olive oil
1	teaspoon almond extract
½	teaspoon pure vanilla extract

Topping:

| 2 | tablespoons fruit-only raspberry jam or another berry jam |
| 2 | tablespoons sliced almonds |

Preheat oven to 350°. Lightly oil an 8-inch square pan. In a large bowl combine oats, oat bran, and baking powder. Mix well. In another bowl, combine remaining ingredients. Add to oat mixture and mix well. Let stand 10 minutes. Stir mixture and spread into pan. Smooth the top. Bake 35 minutes. Cool in pan. Spread jam evenly over top of cooled cake. Sprinkle with almonds. Cut into bars, serve warm or cold.

Gingersnaps

¾	cup whole wheat flour (finely sifted)
¼	cup oat bran
1	teaspoon baking soda
½	teaspoon ground ginger
¼	teaspoon ground cinnamon
⅓	teaspoon ground cloves
¼	cup molasses
2	tablespoons olive oil
1	teaspoon pure vanilla extract
2	tablespoons water

Preheat oven to 375°. Lightly oil a baking sheet. In large bowl combine finely sifted flour, oat bran, baking soda, and spices and mix well. In a small bowl combine remaining ingredients. Add to dry mixture and mix well. Break off pieces of dough and roll into 25 one-inch balls. Place on prepared baking sheet 1½ inches apart. Place a sheet of waxed paper over the cookies and flatten them to ¼-inch thick, using a rolling pin or bottom of a glass. Carefully remove waxed paper. Bake 10–12 minutes. Remove to rack to cool.

Carob Chip Cookies

2½	cups whole wheat flour (finely sifted)
½	teaspoon baking soda
½	cup honey
¼–½	cup olive oil
2	egg whites or 1 egg
1	teaspoon pure vanilla extract
1	cup carob chips
½	cup chopped walnuts

Preheat oven to 375° and lightly oil a cookie sheet.

In a bowl mix finely sifted flour and baking soda. In another bowl mix honey, olive oil, egg whites, and vanilla and mix well.

Mix wet ingredients with the dry ones. Add carob chips and walnuts.

With wet hands roll dough into a desired-size ball, place on cookie sheet. Place a sheet of waxed paper over the cookie balls and press down with the bottom of a glass to flatten (¼-inch thickness) Bake for 10–15 minutes.

Molasses Cookies

1	cup whole wheat flour (finely sifted)
½	cup oat bran
1½	teaspoons baking soda
½	teaspoon ground cinnamon
¼	teaspoon ground nutmeg
	Pinch of ground allspice
	Pinch of ground cloves
3	tablespoons chopped walnuts (optional)
⅓	cup raisins (optional)
3	tablespoons olive oil
¼	cup plus 2 tablespoons molasses
3	tablespoons orange juice
1	teaspoon pure vanilla extract

Preheat oven to 375°. Lightly oil a baking sheet. In large bowl combine finely sifted flour, oat bran, baking soda, and spices and mix well. Add walnuts and raisins. In a small bowl combine remaining ingredients. Add to dry mixture and mix well.

Break off pieces of dough and roll into 36 balls. Place on prepared baking sheet. Place a sheet of waxed paper over cookies and flatten them to ¼-inch thick, using a rolling pin or the bottom of a glass. Carefully remove waxed paper. Bake 10 to 15 minutes. Remove to wire rack to cool.

Banana-Oatmeal Cookies

1	cup whole wheat flour (finely sifted)
1	cup rolled oats

½   teaspoon baking soda
½   teaspoon ground cinnamon
¼   teaspoon ground nutmeg
3   tablespoons chopped pecans
3   tablespoons olive oil
¼   cup honey
½   cup mashed ripe banana
1   teaspoon pure vanilla extract
⅛   cup water

Preheat oven to 375°. Lightly oil a baking sheet. In large bowl combine finely sifted flour, oats, baking soda, spices, and pecans, and mix well. In a small bowl combine remaining ingredients. Add to dry mixture and mix well. Drop mixture by rounded teaspoonfuls onto baking sheet. Bake 10–15 minutes. Remove to a wire rack to cool.

Peanut Oatmeal Cookies

1½   cups rolled oats
½–¾   cup whole wheat flour (finely sifted)
1   teaspoon baking powder
1   teaspoon ground cinnamon
¼   cup honey
¼   cup chopped peanuts (unsalted)
¼   cup raisins
½   cup applesauce
½   cup apple juice
2   tablespoons olive oil
1   teaspoon pure vanilla extract

In a large bowl combine oats, finely sifted flour, baking powder, and cinnamon. In a small bowl combine remaining ingredients. Add to oat mixture and mix well. Let stand for 10 minutes.

Preheat oven to 375°. Lightly oil a baking sheet. Stir batter once, then drop by level tablespoonfuls onto prepared baking sheet. Bake 15 minutes. Remove to a wire rack to cool.

Oatmeal Cookies

1½	cups rolled oats
½–¾	cup whole wheat flour (finely sifted)
1	teaspoon baking powder
1	teaspoon ground cinnamon
¼	cup honey
¼	cup chopped peanuts (unsalted)
¼	cup raisins
½	cup applesauce
½	cup apple juice
2	tablespoons olive oil
1	teaspoon pure vanilla

In a large bowl combine oats, finely sifted flour, baking powder, and cinnamon. In a small bowl combine remaining ingredients. Add to oat mixture and mix well. Let stand for 10 minutes. Preheat oven to 375°. Lightly oil a baking sheet. Stir batter once, then drop by level tablespoonfuls onto prepared baking sheet. Bake 15 minutes. Remove to a wire rack to cool.

Strawberry & Banana Dessert

6	ounces extra-firm tofu
12	ounces silken-firm tofu
2	tablespoons pure maple syrup
2	tablespoons honey
½	teaspoon pure vanilla
12	ounces fresh or frozen strawberries
1	large extra-ripe banana

Place all ingredients into a blender or food processor. Blend until very smooth. Chill—it will set. Serve with fresh fruit or as a pie filling.

Strawberry Ice Cream

16	ounces frozen or fresh strawberries
2	cups of oat, soy, rice, or almond milk

1   teaspoon pure vanilla extract
1   teaspoon honey

Pour all ingredients into a blender and blend until smooth (should be very thick). Pour into container to be frozen for several hours. Very yummy!

Carob Brownies

¾   cup whole wheat flour (finely sifted)
¾   cup oat bran
¼   cup carob powder
1   teaspoon baking powder
1   teaspoon baking soda
2   egg whites or 1 egg
½   cup pure maple syrup
3   tablespoons olive oil
½   cup apple juice
½   cup applesauce (unsweetened)
2   teaspoons pure vanilla extract
¼   teaspoon almond extract
2½   tablespoons chopped walnuts
2½   tablespoons carob chips

Preheat oven to 350°. Lightly oil an 8-inch baking pan. Mix all dry ingredients, excluding walnuts and carob chips, in a bowl. Blend all wet ingredients in a blender, and then add to dry ingredients. Mix well. Fold in walnuts and carob chips. Place into prepared pan. Bake 40 minutes. Cool in pan and cut into squares before serving.

Pound Cake

2   cups whole wheat flour (finely sifted)
½   cup oat bran
½   cup rolled oats
2   teaspoons baking powder
1   teaspoon baking soda

2	teaspoons ground cinnamon
1	teaspoon ground nutmeg
¼	cup chopped walnuts
½	cup honey
¼	cup olive oil
1	cup apple juice
1	tablespoon pure vanilla extract
4	egg whites or 3 egg whites plus 1 whole egg
1	large apple, unpeeled, chopped
1	large pear, unpeeled, chopped
½	cup raisins

Preheat oven to 350°. Lightly spray a 10-inch tube pan with olive oil. In a large bowl combine finely sifted flour, oat bran, rolled oats, baking powder, baking soda, cinnamon, nutmeg, and nuts. Mix well. In another bowl combine honey, oil, apple juice, vanilla, and eggs. Beat with a fork or whisk until blended. Add to dry ingredients along with apple, pear, and raisins. Mix well. Spoon into prepared pan. Bake 45 minutes. Cool in pan 5 minutes and remove to a wire rack to cool.

Sunflower Seed Crackers

Makes 72 small crackers. Prep time: 15 min. Cooking time: 30 min.

1	cup raw, unshelled sunflower seeds
½	cup sesame seeds
½	teaspoon salt or herbamare
¼	cup water

Preheat oven to 325°. Grind seeds in a food processor to a fine meal. Add the sesame seeds and salt and pulse until just combined. Add the water and pulse to mix. Take a cookie sheet and cover with baking parchment. Spread the dough onto the parchment and cover the top with another piece of parchment. Press the dough into a thin sheet (but no holes). Peel off the top layer and score into squares with a pizza cutter. Bake for 30 minutes or until golden. Allow to cool. Break along the scored lines.

Nutritional Analysis per Serving: Calories: 20, Carbs: 1g, Fat: 1g, Protein: 1g

Dessert Nut Balls

Makes 30 servings. Prep time: 10 min.

1	small jar nut butter (organic peanut butter or almond)
½	cup raisins or other dried fruit
½	cup seeds (flax, sunflower, pumpkin, etc.)
⅓	cup honey
¼	cup shredded, unsweetened coconut (will need more to roll the balls in)
¼	cup cocoa powder *(optional)* (This is to make them chocolate flavored.)

Process all of the above ingredients in a food processor until smooth. Take the paste and roll into 2-inch balls. Roll the balls in extra coconut. Refrigerate or freeze in baggies.

Can add other baking extracts for different flavors such as: butterscotch, amaretto, peppermint, etc.

Serving size: One or two—these balls are high in calories so only one or two should be eaten. They are a nice complement to a vegetable or fruit snack.

No-Bake Cookies

Makes 20 servings. Prep time: 5 min. Cooking time: 5 min.

This is a much-healthier version of the traditional recipe.

¼	cup butter
¼	cup coconut oil
½	cup milk or milk substitute (rice, almond, oat milk)
⅓	cup sugar (traditional recipes call for 2 cups, which makes it sickeningly sweet)
¼	cup cocoa
1	teaspoon vanilla
	Pinch of salt
1½	cups quick oats
1½	cups shredded, unsweetened coconut

Melt butter and coconut oil in the saucepan. Add milk, sugar, cocoa, vanilla, and salt and bring to a boil for 30 seconds, stirring rapidly. Remove from the burner, add oats and coconut. When cooled, form into small balls, refrigerate.

Smoothie

Makes 2 servings. Prep time: 5 min.

1	cup milk or milk substitute
½	cup water
1	organic raw egg
1	scoop Berry Living Fuel™
⅔	cup frozen berries
2	tablespoons shredded, unsweetened coconut
6	almonds, soaked overnight

Add ingredients to a high-powered blender and blend on low at first and then increase to high until smooth. If you have a Vitamix (www.vitamix.com), you can sneak chunks of bland vegetables into the smoothie without the kids knowing (cucumber, celery, green cabbage, etc.).

Nutritional Analysis per Serving: Calories: 360, Carbs: 14g, Fat: 18.6g, Protein: 20g

Chocolate Shake

Makes 1 serving. Prep time: 5 min.

1	cup milk
1	tablespoon peanut butter
⅔	cup frozen berries
1–2	organic raw eggs and/OR 1 scoop protein powder like Living Fuel™
1	tablespoon cocoa powder
2	cups ice cubes
¼	teaspoon Stevia if your kids like it (not needed if using Living Fuel)

Add ingredients to a blender and blend on low at first and then increase to high until smooth.

Nutritional Analysis per Serving: Calories: 350, Carbs: 23g, Fat: 16g, Protein: 20g

NOTES

INTRODUCTION: EXCELLING IN AN AVERAGE WORLD

1. April 30, 2006, World Health Organization (WHO), foodingredients.com.
2. "FDA Puts Warning on ADHD Drugs," *USA Today*, Feb. 19 2006. Childhood Obesity Prevention Study, Institute of Medicine of the National Academies, September 2004; drawn from *Preventing Childhood Obesity: Health in the Balance*, 2005, Institute of Medicine, www.iom.edu.
3. Ibid.
4. Ibid.
5. Ibid.
6. Ibid.
7. "Media Use Among Children By Age," Source: Roberts, et al., 1999. Henry J. Kaiser Foundation (used in the Institute of Medicine's Childhood Obesity Study).
8. Gary Taubes, "What If It's All Been a Big Fat Lie?" *New York Times*, July 7, 2002. Located on www.mercola.com with comments from Dr. Mercola.
9. Ibid.
10. FDA Puts Warning on ADHD Drugs, USA Today, Feb. 19 2006
11. Salynn Boyles, WebMD Medical News, Reviewed By Michael Smith, MD, April 14, 2005.
12. Parenthood.com, Debra Gordaon.
13. www.webmd.com/content/article/23/1728_57268.htm.
14. Lori Ann Navarrete, "Melancholy in the Millennium: A Study of Depression Among Adolescents with and without Learning Disabilities," High School Journal 82, no. 3 (Feb/March 1999): 137.
15. "Mental Illness: More Children are on Prescription Drugs for Psychiatric Disorders," Mental Health Weekly Digest (Jan. 03).
16. Combined annual meeting of the Pediatric Academic Societies and the American Academy of Pediatrics, May 19, 2000.

17. www.mercola.com, Dr. Mercola's comments to article "Each Daily Soda Increases Obesity Risk 60%, *The Lancet* 2/28/2001;357:505-508.
18. Carol Torgan, Ph.D., "Childhood Obesity on the Rise," *NIH Word on Health*, June 2002.
19. Gary Taubes, "What If It's All Been a Big Fat Lie?"

CHAPTER 1: CONFESSIONS OF A TWINKIE-EATING TV JUNKIE

1. Ben Lerner, *Body by God* (Thomas Nelson, 2003). It is also cited on www.mercola.com in an article titled "Is the Wellness Revolution Really Working?" by Dr. Ben Lerner, with comments from Dr. Mercola.
2. Ibid.
3. Ibid.

CHAPTER 2: WHY PEER INFLUENCE IS SO POWERFUL

1. Em Twoey, *Proteen: A Positive Approach to Understanding Adolescents* (Cleveland, TN: Pathway Press, 2002), 21–33.

CHAPTER 3: JUNK-FOOD NATION

1. Dr. Joseph Mercola with Rachael Droege, "Four Ways Junk Food Marketing Targets Your Kids," http://www.mercola.com/2003/nov/26/junk_food_marketing.htm.
2. Sarah Ellison, "Companies Fight for Right to Plug Kids' Food," *Wall Street Journal*, January 26, 2005.
3. Mercola and Droege, "Four Ways Junk Food Marketing Targets Your Kids."
4. *New York Times*, April 6, 2006, http://www.nytimes.com/2006/04/06/education06 lunch.html?ex=1147320000&en=964e1ad45762b579&ei=5070.
5. *Washington Post*, February 27, 2001, Page A01.
6. ABC News, July 27, 2004.
7. http://www.surgeongeneral.gov/news/testimony/reshapinghealthcare10012003.
8. *Washington Post*, December 14, 2001, Page A03.
9. Annual Experimental Biology 2002 Conference, New Orleans, LA, April 22, 2002.
10. Eric Schlosser, *Fast Food Nation* (Houghton Mifflin, 2001).
11. *New England Journal of Medicine*, January 1, 1998;338:52–54.
12. http://harkin.senate.gov/news.cfm?id=222885.
13. www.panaonline.org.
14. Childhood Obesity Prevention Study, Institute of Medicine of the National Academies, September 2004; drawn from *Preventing Childhood Obesity: Health in the Balance*, 2005, Institute of Medicine, www.iom.edu.
15. http://www.panaonline.org
16. Ibid.
17. "Chicago Group Tackles Childhood Obesity," Associated Press, October 18, 2004.
18. www.subway.com/Publishing/PubRelations/PressRelease/pr071404-1.pdf.

19. *NeuroImage*, April 2004.
20. Ibid.

CHAPTER 4: HOW THE BODY GAINS—AND LOSES—FAT

1. "Insulin Resistance Rampant Among Overweight Children," Annual Scientific Sessions of the American Heart Association, November 2000, New Orleans, La.
2. Mercola, Joseph, *Dr. Mercola's Total Health Program.*
3. Experimental Biology Conference April 2005, http://www.scienceblog.com/cms/node/8028.
4. Mercola.
5. "Low-Carb Stores Becoming More Common," *USA Today*, August 19, 2003.
6. "Restaurants Cashing in on Low Carb," *New York Times*, January 4, 2004.
7. Mercola.
8. Second-opinions.co.uk.

CHAPTER 5: THE HEALTH AND FITNESS ZONE

1. Dr. Joseph Mercola with Alison Rose Levy, *The No-Grain Diet* (New York: Dutton, 2003), 19–20.
2. Ibid.

CHAPTER 6: THE RIGHT FOODS: HIGH-OCTANE FUEL FOR YOUR CHILD

1. www.mercola.com, "Nearly 2 Billion Are Overweight or Obese," *Reuters Health,* March 17 2003, with Dr. Mercola's comments.
2. Dr. Joseph Mercola, *Dr. Mercola's Total Health Program*
3. Study: "Obesity Impairs Immune Response of Mice, Boosts Chances of Dying from Influenza Infection"; University of North Carolina at Chapel Hill School of Medicine, 4/4/05, http://news.biocompare.com/newsstory.asp?id=73796.
4. Mercola.

CHAPTER 8: LIQUID ASSETS: THE GOOD, BAD, AND UGLY OF BEVERAGES

1. *The Lancet*, 2001, 357:505–508.

CHAPTER 9: ARE SUPPLEMENTS ALL THEY'RE CRACKED UP TO BE?

1. L. Troppmann, K. Gray-Donald, and T. Johns, "Supplement Use: Is There Any Nutritional Benefit?" *Journal of the American Dietetic Association*, June 2002; 102:818-825, http://www.ncbi.nlm.nih.gov/entrez/query.fcgi?cmd=Retrieve&db=PubMed&list_uids=12067048&dopt=Abstract.
2. Cancerpage.com, January 6, 2005; American Dietetic Association, Dec. 28, 2004.
3. "Wal-Mart Eyes Organic Foods, and Brand Names Get in Line," *New York Times*, May 12, 2006.
4. National Academy of Sciences Committee on Scientific and Regulatory Issues Underlying Pesticide Use Patterns and Agricultural Innovation, National Research

Council Regulating Pesticides in Food: The Delaney Paradox 1987 http://www.nap.edu/catalog/1013.html.

5. B. Baker, C. M. Benbrook, E. Groth, et al., "Pesticide residues in conventional, IPMgrown and organic foods: Insights from three U.S. data sets," *Food Additives and Contaminants*, vol. 19, no. 5, May 2002, 427–446 http://www.consumersunion.org/food/organicsumm.htm.

6. Environmental Working Group http://www.foodnews.org/reportcard.php.

7. Ibid.

CHAPTER 10: MAKING CHANGES THAT STICK

1. *Journal of Clinical Endocrinology & Metabolism*, August 2001; 86:3787–3794.

CHAPTER 11: GET MOVING!

1. *Tallahassee Democrat*, October 28, 2004.

2. K. B. Blomquist and F. Danner (1987). Effects of physical conditioning on information-processing efficiency, Percept. Mot. Skills 65 175–186.

3. J. J. Keays, K. R. Allison (1995). The effects of regular moderate to vigorous physical activity on student outcomes; Can J Public h Health 1995 Jan–Feb; 86(1): 62–65.

4. D. Reynolds, R. I. Nicolson, H. Hambly, Evaluation of an exercise-based treatment for children with reading difficulties, *Dyslexia* 2003 Feb.; 9(1) 48–71 (discussion, 46–47).

5. Ibid.

6. R. D. Hill et al. (1993). The impact of long-term exercise training on psychological function in older adults; J. Gerontol. 48: 12–17. L. F. Berkman et al., High, usual and impaired functioning in community-dwelling older men and women: findings from the MacArthur Foundation Research Network on Successful Aging; J. Clin. Epidemiol 46 (1993) 1129–1140.

7. D. Laurin et al. (2001). Physical activity and risk of cognitive impairment and dementia in elderly persons; Arch Neurol. 58: 498–504.

8. C. Frabre et al. (2002). Improvement of cognitive function by mental and/or individualized aerobic training in healthy elderly subjects; Int J Sports Med 23 (6): 425–421; J. Etnier et al. (1999). The relationships among pulmonary function, aerobic fitness and cognitive functioning in older COPD patients; Chest 116 (4): 953–960.

9. P. D. Tomporowski (2003). Effects of acute bouts of exercise on cognition; Acta Psychol 112 (3): 297–324.

10. C. W. Cotman and N. C. Berchtold (2002). Exercise: a behavioral intervention to enhance brain health and plasticity; Trends in Neurosci 25 (6) p. 295–301.

11. W. Stummer et al. (1994). Reduced mortality and brain damage after locomoter activity in gerbil forebrain ischemia; Stroke 25: 1862–1896.

12. E. Carro et al. (2001). Circulating insulin-like growth factor I mediates the protective effects of physical exercise against brain insults of different etiology and anatomy; J. Neurosci 21: 5678–5684.

13. K. R. Isaacs et al. (1992). Exercise and the brain: angiogenesis in the adult rat cerebellum after vigorous physical activity and motor skill learning; J. Cereb Blood Flow Metab 12: 110–119.

14. H. van Praag et al. (1999). Running enhances neurogenesis, learning and long-term potentiation in mice; Proc Natl. Acad Sci USA 96: 13427–13431.

15. N. C. Berchtold et al. (2002), Hippocampal brain-derived neurotrophic factor gene regulation by exercise and the medial septum, *J. Neurosci Res* 68 (5): 511–521; A. Russo-Neustadt et al. (1999), Physical activity-antidepressant treatment combination: impact on BDNF and behavior in an animal model, *Behavi Brain Res* 120 10: 87–95; E. Carro et al., Circulating insulin-like growth factor I mediates effects of exercise on the brain, J Neurosci 20 (2000) p. 2926-2933.

16. "PE Gets Benched," Associated Press, January 18, 2005.

ABOUT THE AUTHORS

Dr. Joseph Mercola is trained as a family physician but now focuses exclusively in natural medicine education. He has been interviewed by the major television networks and dozens of nationally broadcast radio shows. His Web site, www.mercola.com, is the leading natural health site on the Internet.

Dr. Ben Lerner was an academic all-American wrestler in college and has served as a Chiropractor, nutritionist, and fitness trainer for the U.S. wrestling teams in six World Championships and two Olympics. His breakthrough strategies for total health and well-being are the foundation for the Maximized Living Mentor program and the thriving Centers for Maximized Living, which he helps open and operate all throughout the U.S. (www.maximizedliving.com)